SOCIAL MURDER

Austerity and Life Expec
in the UK

David Walsh and Gerry McCartney

P

First published in Great Britain in 2025 by

Policy Press, an imprint of
Bristol University Press
University of Bristol
1–9 Old Park Hill
Bristol
BS2 8BB
UK
t: +44 (0)117 374 6645
e: bup-info@bristol.ac.uk

Details of international sales and distribution partners are available at policy.bristoluniversitypress.co.uk

British Library Cataloguing in Publication Data
A catalogue record for this book is available from the British Library

ISBN 978-1-4473-7307-0 hardcover
ISBN 978-1-4473-7308-7 paperback
ISBN 978-1-4473-7309-4 ePub
ISBN 978-1-4473-7310-0 ePdf

Cover design: Nicky Borowiec
Front cover image: © Adobestock/jozefmicic

This book is dedicated to all those, and the families of those, affected by the policies of austerity

When one individual inflicts bodily injury upon another such injury that death results, we call the deed manslaughter; when the assailant knew in advance that the injury would be fatal, we call his deed murder. But when society places hundreds ... in such a position that they inevitably meet a too early and an unnatural death ... when it deprives thousands of the necessaries of life, places them under conditions in which they cannot live ... its deed is murder just as surely as the deed of the single individual; disguised, malicious murder, murder against which none can defend himself, which does not seem what it is, because no man sees the murderer, because the death of the victim seems a natural one, since the offence is more one of omission than of commission. But murder it remains ... social murder.[1]

Friedrich Engels, The Condition of the
Working Class in England, 1845

Over 170 years after Engels, Britain is still a country that murders its poor.[2]

Aditya Chakrabortty, in reference to the
Grenfell fire, The Guardian, 2017

The shift towards austerity [has] also legitimised the use of economic violence against disabled people, and other groups deemed 'unproductive' by the ruling class. In the UK ... [it] would not be an exaggeration to describe some of these cases ... as social murder.[3]

Grace Blakely,
Tribune Magazine, 2023

Contents

List of figures and tables

Figures

Tables

About the authors

David Walsh is Senior Lecturer in Health Inequalities at the University of Glasgow, and previously Programme Manager at the Glasgow Centre for Population Health.

Gerry McCartney is Professor of Wellbeing Economy at the University of Glasgow and Honorary Consultant in Public Health at Public Health Scotland.

Acknowledgements

We are enormously grateful to all those who helped us with this endeavour.

First and foremost, our heartfelt thanks go to the relatives of some of the people featured in the book both for allowing us to use their loved ones' stories and for the additional insights that they were able to provide: Anne-Marie O'Sullivan (daughter of Michael), Gill Thompson (sister of David Clapson) and Nicole Drury (daughter of Moira). We are also grateful to Patrick Butler, Amelia Gentleman and Karen McVeigh from *The Guardian* newspaper, and John Pring from the Disability News Service, for help in putting us in touch with Anne-Marie, Gill and Nicole.

Thank you also to *The Guardian* journalist Frances Ryan for permission to use the stories of Paul and Rachel, and also to Saket Priyadarshi and, especially, Natasha Devereux for invaluable help with Ellen's story.

Please note that the additional research for the book was approved by the University of Glasgow College of Social Sciences Research Ethics Committee (application no. 400220358).

Grateful thanks also to those who provided helpful material for, and/or checked sections of, the book: Tina Beattie at Sheffield-Hallam University, Berengere Chabanis and Jennie Coyle at the Glasgow Centre for Population Health, Howard Reed of Landman Economics, David Webster at Glasgow University, as well as Maria Teresa de Haro Moro, Rosalia Munoz-Arroyo, Lauren Schofield and Martin Taulbut (all at Public Health Scotland). In a similar vein, thank you to our co-authors of the 2022 report, 'Resetting the course for population health', which features prominently here: Lynda Fenton and Rebecca Devine.

A broader set of thanks are due to all our co-authors of the various reports and journal articles that we cite, including: Tina Beattie, Phil Broadbent, Alberto Ciancio, Ruth Dundas, Lynda Fenton, Colin Fischbacher, Eilidh Fletcher, Thierry Gagné, Christine Gallagher, Marcia Gibson, Vittal Katikireddi, Maria Kaye-Bardgett, Kirsty Little, Bob McMaster, Jon Minton, Jane Parkinson, Frank Popham, Eugenio Proto, Andy Pulford, Julie Ramsay, Liz Richardson, Mark Robinson, Rosie Seaman, Debs Shipton, Martin Taulbut, Bruce Whyte, Grant Wyper and Anwen Zhang .

We also grateful to everyone at Policy Press, especially Laura Vickers-Rendall and Isobel Bainton, as well as to the anonymous reviewers who provided helpful comments.

Finally, thanks to our employers at the time of writing for giving us the opportunity to write the book in regular working hours – the Glasgow Centre for Population Health and the University of Glasgow.

Please note that all royalties from the sale of this book go to the NHS, and not to the authors.

Authors' note

The seven individual stories included in this book – those of Michael, Rachel, Frances, Paul, Moira, Ellen and David – were selected in an attempt to illustrate the impacts of different facets of the UK Government's austerity policies on individual people: 'work capability assessments' (Michael); cuts to social care services (Rachel); the bedroom tax (Frances); cuts to housing services (Paul); changes to social security and their impact on mental health (Moira), and on people who use drugs (Ellen); and social security 'sanctions' (David).

Their stories come from different sources. Michael's, Moira's and David's stories were originally highlighted by journalists in different media articles (all of which we have cited accordingly). We were additionally able to provide further details through discussion (via e-mails or online meetings) with family members, to whom we are enormously grateful (and whom we list in the acknowledgements section of the book). Frances's story was also covered in appropriately cited media articles.

Ellen's story was provided by one of the social workers who worked with her. Ellen is not her real name and no identifiable information is included in her story.

Finally, Rachel's and Paul's stories were originally included in *The Guardian* journalist Frances Ryan's excellent book, *Crippled: Austerity and the Demonisation of Disabled People*. We are grateful to Frances, and her publisher, for permission to retell these important stories here.

Michael

Michael O'Sullivan was born in 1953 in the small market town of Listowel, in County Kerry in southern Ireland. In the mid-1970s he followed the well-trodden path to London in search of employment. There he worked as a builder, and in the trade was known as a highly practical man: on building sites, Mickey (as he was known to workmates) was the man who could resolve a problem, the man who would find the solution. One of his employers described him as a 'genius' when it came to all manner of building tasks: he could turn his hand to anything, and his answer was always 'no problem' when asked to find a way to get something difficult done.[1]

Not long after moving to London, he met (at the Mecca for the London Irish at the time, the Galtymore dance hall in Cricklewood) and married his wife, and settled down to work and family life. He is described by his daughter, Anne-Marie, as being 'tall, dark and handsome', very kind in nature, but also shy and nervous. He doted on his family and, living in Highgate, he liked to take long walks on nearby Hampstead Heath, as it reminded him of home. But by the time he was in his late 40s, a variety of mental health issues meant he could no longer work: he would eventually be diagnosed by a psychiatrist and clinical psychologist as having recurrent depression, panic attacks linked to agoraphobia, and severe anxiety issues. In 2000, he was signed off work and received sickness benefit from the state.[2,3]

In 2010 a raft of new policies were introduced by the UK's Conservative-Liberal Democrat coalition government which included a greater focus on assessing whether people who, like Michael, were on sickness benefits were in fact capable of working.[4,5] This was part of a package of measures aimed at saving money – the intention was to cut the social security budget by tens of billions of pounds over the following decade.[6] ATOS, a multinational information technology (IT) company, held the contract to undertake these medical assessments. The company employed people with different levels of health qualifications to do this, and there were concerns that staff were under pressure to declare people fit for work so that they could then be taken off sickness benefit.[7,8] There were also suggestions that the ATOS employees were financially incentivised to assess as many people as possible per day.[9]

In August 2012, at the age of 59, Michael was called to attend this 'work capability assessment'. It lasted 12 minutes. In that time an ATOS-employed physiotherapist decided that Michael was fit to work. He would no longer receive sickness benefit and would have to look for a job.

Increasingly worried about what the future held for him, Michael was sent on a training course to obtain a certificate that would enable him to work on a building site again. In poor mental health, depressed, and with low self-esteem and anxiety issues, he was bullied and humiliated by the much younger trainees. At the end of the first week, utterly desperate and failing to cope, he tried to kill himself. But he survived.

He was subsequently declared unfit for any work by his general practitioner (GP) and moved back onto sickness benefit.

In March the following year, barely four months after attempting suicide, Michael was asked to attend a second work capability assessment. Despite clinical diagnoses of severe mental health problems, and despite still being signed off as unable to work by his GP, he was again declared fit for work by the ATOS-employed health professional. He was taken off sickness benefit and told to find a job. A few months later, on the eve of starting the four-week work placement that had been found for him, Michael hanged himself. He was 60 years old.

On the night he died, his daughter Anne-Marie found five freshly ironed shirts, a hard hat and a pair of new, steel-capped boots all laid out in his bedroom in preparation for the work placement he couldn't face. At the inquest into his death, the coroner, Mary Hassell, stated that his suicide was 'caused by his recent assessment as being fit for work, and his view of the likely consequences of that'.[2]

1

Introduction

Death is a daily part of life. Everyone dies, and everyone has their own stories and experiences of someone's death – a friend, a colleague, a neighbour, a family member. Perhaps even a story like Michael O'Sullivan's. These individual stories are obviously hugely important. But what's also important is what they *add up to*, what these stories mean *collectively*. Because understanding their totality – the circumstances of these deaths, the ages of the people involved, the absolute number that occur over time – tells us a lot: it tells us about the overall health of the population; but more than that, it also tells us about the very nature of the society we live in.

We use lots of such measures of *population health* for this purpose. The age-standardised mortality rate (ASMR) is one of these: this is just the number of deaths per head of population, taking age into account.[10] Life expectancy, a very similar metric, is another. It's worth emphasising that life expectancy is not, as it is sometimes misreported to be, a prediction of how long a baby born today will live in the future. Rather, it's just a reflection of the ages that people are *currently* dying at (or living until). It's simply a different, and arguably more understandable, way of summarising the mortality rate.[11]

Life expectancy data show that in the 1920s men in England and Wales were living, on average, until their mid-50s (Figure 1.1). Nowadays – and again, *on average* – they live around 25 years longer. That's an extraordinary change over a relatively short period of time. It reflects not just better health overall, but the vast societal improvements that underpin it: significantly better living conditions, public health success stories like childhood vaccination programmes, medical and pharmaceutical advances and much more. In the UK, this dramatic period of improvement includes the creation of the modern welfare state in the post-war period: free healthcare through the establishment of the National Health Service (NHS), the introduction of old age pensions for all and greater financial support from the state for those in need. In other words, the creation of a much better, more caring, society compared to what had gone before.

In fact, in the UK life expectancy has increased (and mortality rates have correspondingly decreased[14]) more or less constantly for more than a century. Notably, the only exceptions to this have been times of absolute crisis: world wars and pandemics.[15] This is also true of other European

Figure 1.1: Male and female life expectancy (combined), Scotland and England and Wales, 1900–2019

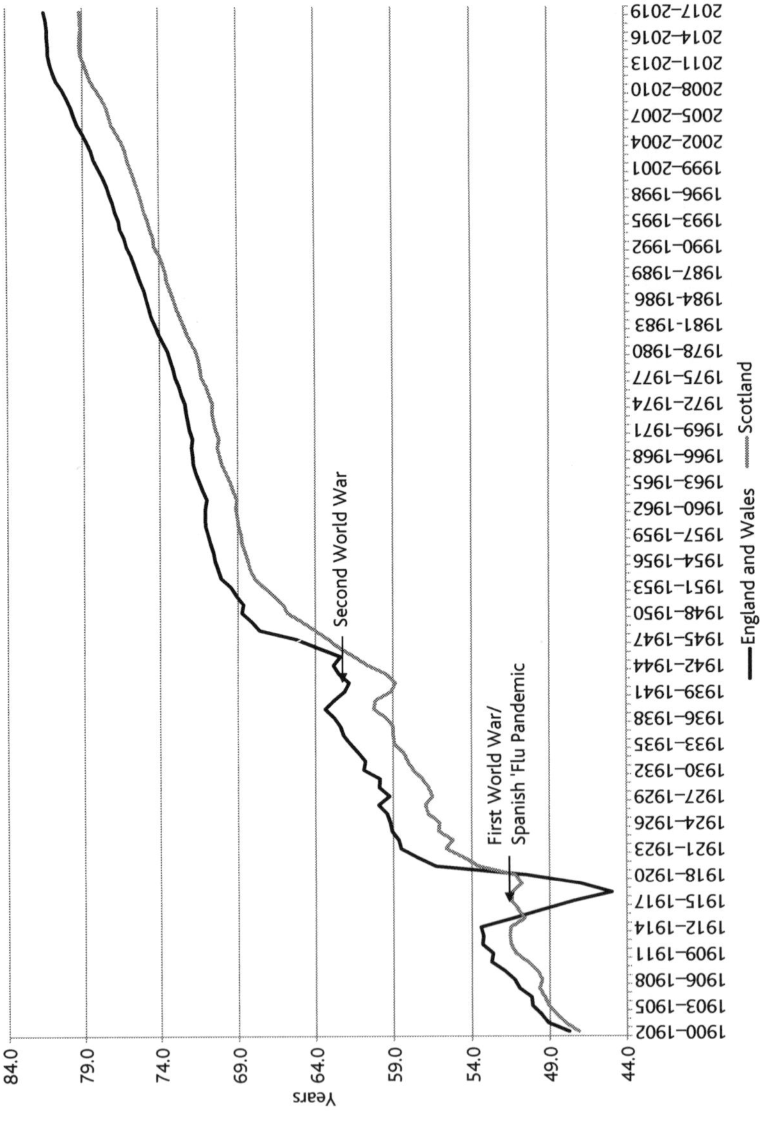

England and Wales ——— Scotland

Notes: Refer to the notes at the end of this book for full description.[13]
Source: Human Mortality Database[12]

Figure 1.2: Life expectancy, males and females, Scotland and England and Wales, 1980–2019

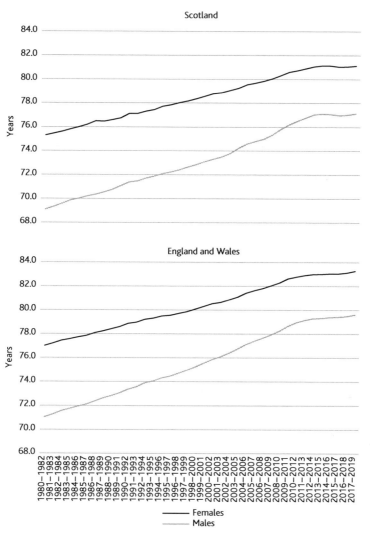

Notes: Refer to the notes at the end of this book for full description.[17]
Source: Human Mortality Database[12]

countries, with the exception of Russia and a small number of other Eastern European countries which suffered falls in life expectancy associated with other significant societal crises as they made a rapid transition to capitalism. Other than those crises, however, average life expectancy – as a marker of overall societal progress – has consistently improved.

It's quite extraordinary, therefore, to state that in the UK around 2012, this all more or less stopped. Following decades of continual improvement, life expectancy suddenly stopped increasing in Scotland, England and Wales

(Figures 1.1 and 1.2) and Northern Ireland. Worse than that, among poorer populations (for example, people living in what are assessed to be the 20 per cent most socioeconomically deprived neighbourhoods of each UK nation) it actually went into reverse: life expectancy declined, and so death rates actually *increased* (Figure 1.3).[16] In some parts of the UK, the change to *premature* mortality rates (death under the age of 65 years) has been nothing short of astonishing: as one example, look at the rates for females living in Glasgow's poorer areas in Figure 1.4. Between 2001 around 2012, the mortality rate dropped sharply, and inequalities (the gap between the rates in the poorest and wealthiest areas of the city) clearly narrowed. However,

Figure 1.3: Age-standardised mortality rates (ASMRs) for females, all ages, Scotland and England and their 20 per cent most and least deprived neighbourhoods, 1981–2019

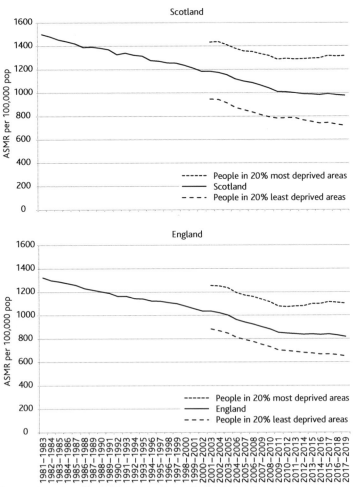

Notes: Refer to the notes at the end of this book for full description.[19]
Source: Walsh & McCartney 2023[18]

Figure 1.4: Age-standardised mortality rates (ASMRs) for females aged 0–64 years, Glasgow and its 20 per cent most and least deprived neighbourhoods, 1981–2021

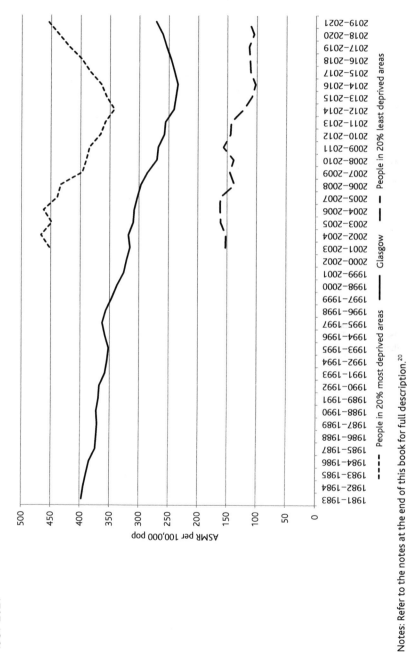

Notes: Refer to the notes at the end of this book for full description.[20]
Source: Walsh and McCartney 2023[18]

a dramatic reversal of that trend means that by 2019/21, death rates were higher than they had been 20 years previously. It's absolutely extraordinary. We'll show further examples of these shocking changes in the next chapter.

All this has been made even worse by the COVID-19 pandemic, which increased death rates further in 2020 and 2021 (also shown in Figure 1.4).

What this means is that in the poorer areas of the UK, in a complete reversal of previous long-term trends, people have been *dying younger*, and dying in greater numbers than before. And overall – across all different parts of the UK – a great many more people have died than should have been the case. Compared to what we expected to happen (based on the previous trends), an estimated additional 335,000 deaths occurred in Scotland, England and Wales between 2012 and 2019.[21] That's a lot more than died directly from COVID-19. Why?

This is a book about evidence. Evidence on the causes of these changed trends from a great many sources, including research teams from across the UK and further afield. And what that evidence shows is that these extraordinary, almost unprecedented, changes to life expectancy and mortality rates have been caused in large part by UK government policies that were implemented from 2010 onwards, and which remain in place today. It is therefore also the story of a scandal, of a tragedy on an enormous scale that did not need to happen.

In the book we will lay out all the evidence of what happened in the UK – what the government did, who was affected by it and how. We will also show what happened in other countries where similar policies were introduced (and in countries where they were not). We'll show how government and national agencies responded to the evidence – and what responses are really needed to address the crisis. In doing all this, we will show further charts of mortality rates, life expectancy and other summary measures of population health. It's important to remember, however, that behind these statistics lie the individual stories of an extraordinary number of people who died before their time. People like Michael O'Sullivan. And others like him whose stories we also share here.

Rachel

Malnutrition is the kind of health problem that we associate with famine and drought in poorer countries, or perhaps with poverty and destitution in Britain way back in Victorian times.

Yet 21st-century Britain is now seeing cases of malnutrition not caused by some rare disease or condition, but due to cuts in social care services. Around 11,000 people were admitted to hospital in England in 2022 with malnutrition,[1] and hundreds of people every year die in England and Wales with malnutrition mentioned on their death certificate.[2] We're seeing malnutrition in people like Rachel.[3,4]

Rachel has arthritis, lupus and Crohn's disease. Although these health problems cause her substantial pain and suffering, for many years she was able to live independently in the New Forest in the south of England with the help of a social care package provided by her local council.

This all started to change after George Osborne became Chancellor of the Exchequer, following the election of the Conservative-Liberal Democrat government in May 2010. As we discuss in more detail in Chapter 3, austerity cuts to a range of public services were introduced not long afterwards.[5] Among the biggest cuts were those to local authority budgets.[6] The reduction in funding was even greater in the north of England and in more deprived areas, impacting disproportionately on those communities that needed the money the most.[6-8]

Local authorities rely on central government funding for most of their income. They can raise money from council tax and business rates, and by charging for some services, but this is a very small proportion of the money they require. Local authorities were left with few options, and inevitably this meant large cuts to the services they provided for their communities. For those services that they could still maintain, it often meant the introduction of charges, or price increases.

The impact of this for people like Rachel has been all too real. In 2010 the first of the cuts were introduced. The visit from the care worker who helped her to go to bed was stopped, putting her ability to live independently in jeopardy. The eligibility rules for support to keep people's houses clean and their gardens tidy was changed to save money, and people aged under 70 were now excluded. Rachel, and people like her, were left to fend for themselves.

In 2011 the care worker support package that was in place to provide a hot evening meal was also withdrawn, leaving Rachel with only one

45-minute morning visit to help her wash and dress. The social work department advised that additional support could be paid for, but this was prohibitively expensive, particularly for someone unable to work.

As if the cuts to local authority social care weren't enough, Rachel was then transferred to the new, and somewhat ironically named, Personal Independence Payment (PIP). This was promptly cut, leaving her without the means to purchase any social care provision, and thus without any of the support services that had previously allowed her to live happily and independently.

Before long, no hot meals were provided on five out of every seven days, there was no help with showering and Rachel was spending the whole day in her nightwear. When she was feeling stronger she was able to prepare meals which she could then later heat up. But on bad days she was living on bread and fruit. It was the withdrawal of these lifeline services, including the humanity provided by the care workers, that led to Rachel's malnutrition.

Rachel's malnutrition was picked up at a regular visit to her GP, and supplements were provided to help. But it is impossible for her GP to fix, because no medical prescription can substitute for the austerity-driven cuts to the local authority services she relied upon. It begs an obvious question: what kind of a society do we live in where people who are ill have their support withdrawn, and where they are ultimately made sicker?

2

What happened in the UK?

Health statistics represent people with the tears wiped off.
Attributed to Austin Bradford Hill

In the first chapter we highlighted the extraordinary changes to life expectancy and mortality rates that have occurred in the UK since the early 2010s. In this chapter we delve into these unprecedented developments in a little more detail to explain: the scale of the divergence from previous trends; when exactly these changes occurred; who was most affected; what happened to particular causes of death; what the additional impact of the COVID-19 pandemic has been; and what all this means for health inequalities in the UK in the 21st century.

What happened – and what should have happened

As we explained in the last chapter, the changes we have seen since 2012 were preceded by over a hundred years of more or less continual improvement.[1,2] The sole exceptions (the 'less' in 'more or less') were times of profound national crisis. The obvious expectation, therefore, was that these improvements would have continued: as we will explain in later chapters, the changes that we have witnessed are not explained by reaching any kind of 'natural limit' to life expectancy,[3] and other countries saw their life expectancy and mortality rates continue to improve throughout the 2010s. So how does *what should have happened* compare with *what actually happened*?

Figure 2.1, adapted from one of our recent studies,[4] answers this question for mortality rates. The figure shows the *observed* and *predicted* mortality rates for males aged 15–84 years in England between 1981 and 2019.[5] Each dot represents the actual mortality rate in each year, while the solid black line is the so-called 'linear trend' that has been fitted to those rates for the years 1981–2011.[6] By extending that line to cover the years 2012–19, we can predict what the rates in those years would have been *if the previous trend had continued*. This is represented by the dashed part of the line. The divergence from around 2012 – the gap between what happened and what was predicted to happen – is very clear.[7]

Figure 2.2, taken from a different study,[8] presents similar comparisons of observed and predicted trends, but this time for life expectancy. It

Figure 2.1: Observed and predicted age-standardised mortality rates (ASMRs), males aged 15–84 years, England 1981–2019

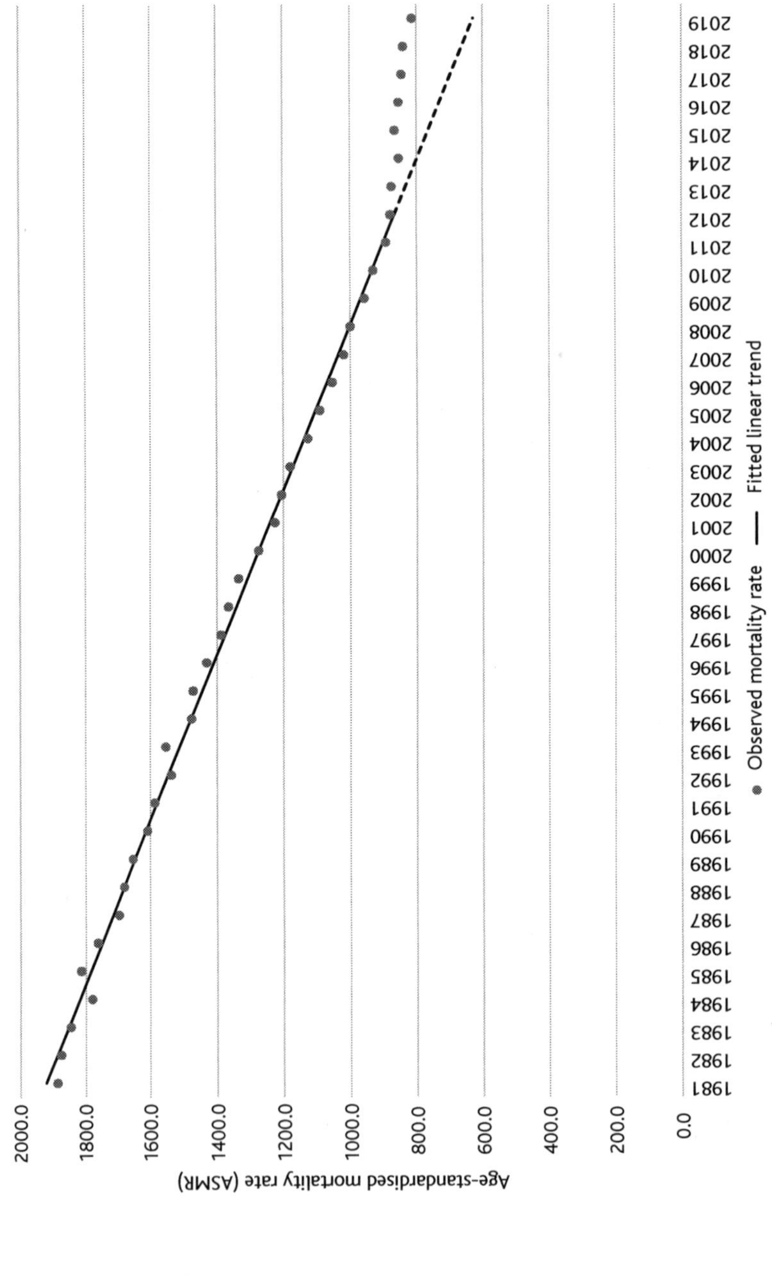

● Observed mortality rate   —— Fitted linear trend

Source: Walsh et al 2022[4]

Figure 2.2: Projected life expectancy trends based on 1990–2011 trends compared with actual life expectancy trends, UK nations, females and males, 2012–18

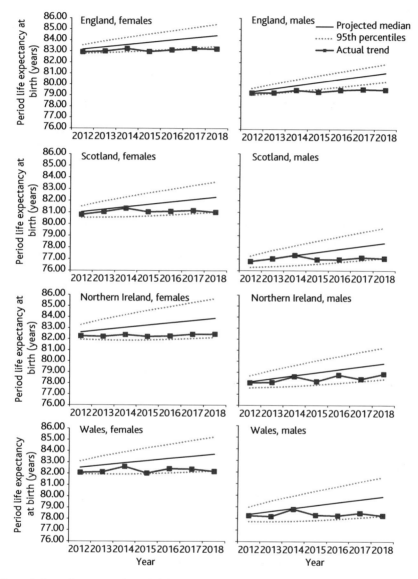

Notes: Refer to the notes at the end of this book for full description.[9]
Source: Minton et al 2020[8]

does so for males and females, and the four constituent nations of the UK. Focusing on the period 2012–18, the widening gap between the projected (black line) and the actual trend (grey line with squares) is clear across all four UK nations.

Another of our studies extended these analyses by estimating what that gap between the predicted and observed mortality rates represented in terms of absolute numbers of deaths[10] – in other words, how many more people died between 2012 and 2019 than should have been the case. The extraordinary overall figure – approximately 335,000 across Scotland, England and Wales – was reported in Chapter 1. The more detailed breakdown supplied in our published journal paper showed that this was comprised of almost 20,000 extra deaths in Scotland and approximately 315,000 in England and Wales. Previously unpublished analyses from the same study showed that the equivalent figure in Northern Ireland was more than 10,000 deaths. That makes a UK total of almost 345,000 additional deaths in the period up to 2019. Other studies have come up with broadly similar numbers.[11,12]

How accurate are these kinds of estimates? On the one hand, as our journal paper made very clear, all sorts of caveats apply to such projections, and the need for cautious interpretation was emphasised. On the other hand, in a sense, the precise number doesn't really matter: whether it's 300,000, 345,000 or 400,000, what matters is that there has been an extraordinary change in the mortality profile of the UK, and a huge number of people have died before their time – in a terrifyingly large number of cases, many, many years before their time. We need to fully understand the details and, especially, the causes of this to make sure it doesn't ever happen again.

When did the trends change?

From looking at Figure 2.1, or indeed any of the four figures included in Chapter 1, it seems pretty obvious when the trends changed – around 2012. You wouldn't think much more work would be required to confirm this, but you'd be wrong: a number of studies have been published in which particular statistical techniques were used to determine exactly when the life expectancy and mortality trends diverged from their previous trajectories.[4,13-15] It's actually important to do this: as mentioned earlier, rates can fluctuate from year to year, and so providing robust statistical evidence that trends have indeed changed is imperative. And more than that, pinpointing the exact year or years is vital when it comes to identifying and understanding the causes.

All that said, the results of those more sophisticated statistical analyses turned out to be basically the same as what Figure 2.1, and the charts in Chapter 1, all imply. The results varied very slightly across different analyses and depending on the particular population groups examined, but the overall answer (expressed in not very statistical language) was indeed: *around 2012*. We'll come back to the significance of that in the next chapter.

Who was most affected?

Income

As already outlined in the opening chapter, at the heart of this whole story are the astonishing changes in death rates among poorer populations that have been seen across the UK. Rates have not only stopped improving, they have gone into reverse. Evidence for females of all ages in Scotland and England was presented in Chapter 1. The same data, but presently slightly differently[16] and alongside rates for males, are shown in Figure 2.3. The trends for premature death (defined here as death under the age of 65 years) are even more shocking. The dramatic reversal of previously sharply falling premature death rates among females in Glasgow was shown in Chapter 1; but we can show similarly dramatic changes across many cities of the UK – a selection is shown in Figure 2.4. Male premature death rates in the poorer parts of Leeds, Liverpool, Bristol and Sheffield all fell between 2001 and around 2010/12, but then – remarkably – started to increase.

There is a wealth of published evidence which shows, using different analytical techniques, these remarkable – and awful – changes that have occurred across the poorer parts of the UK.[10,17,20–24] Examining all this evidence in its entirety, it's worth reflecting on a couple of important issues. First, what do we mean by the 'poorer parts' of the UK? In the country-level analyses such as those shown in Figure 2.3, data are shown for the 20 per cent most socioeconomically deprived neighbourhoods.[25] So these are not trends for the 1 per cent or 2 per cent most deprived – those living on the extremes. These are data for *one fifth of the whole population of England* and *one fifth of the whole population of Scotland*. Second, these changes have obviously taken place in one of the richest countries on earth. With so many years' talk of austerity, food banks, the cost-of-living crisis and all the rest, it can perhaps be easy to forget this. But, by any standard international measure, the UK is very wealthy society;[26] it's just that that wealth is extraordinarily unevenly distributed.[27,28] And in such a wealthy society, we simply shouldn't be seeing these trends at all.

Age, sex and cause of death

Alongside this socioeconomic evidence, an understanding of which sex and age groups have been most affected, and which individual causes of death have seen the most changes, is also hugely important. A considerable amount of research into this has been undertaken,[21,29,30] but it can be succinctly summarised as follows: the changes to mortality rates have been seen for both males and females, all age groups and virtually all causes of death.

Let's explore this in a little more detail. In terms of sex, there is some evidence that, among people living in more deprived areas, mortality

Figure 2.3: Age-standardised mortality rates (ASMRs) 1981–2019, males and females of all ages, Scotland and England and their respective 20 per cent most and least socioeconomically deprived populations

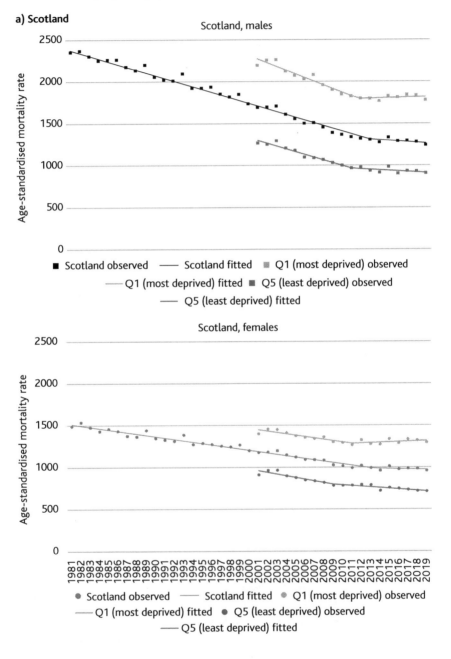

Figure 2.3: Age-standardised mortality rates (ASMRs) 1981–2019, males and females of all ages, Scotland and England and their respective 20 per cent most and least socioeconomically deprived populations (continued)

b) England

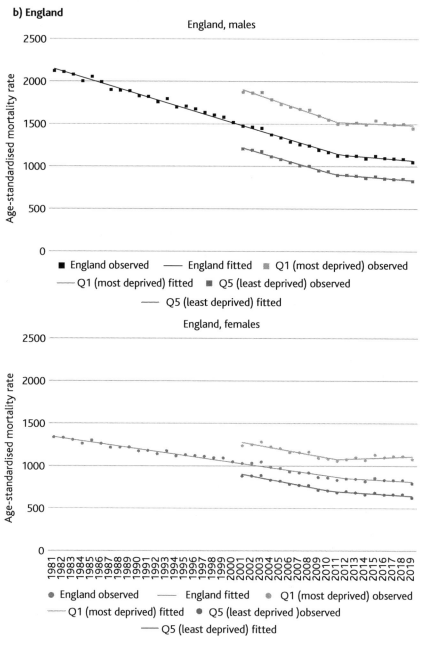

Notes: Refer to the notes at the end of this book for full description.[18]
Source: Walsh and McCartney 2023[17]

Figure 2.4: Age-standardised mortality rates (ASMRs) for males aged 0–64 years, for four English cities and their 20 per cent most and least deprived neighbourhoods, 1981–2019

a) Leeds

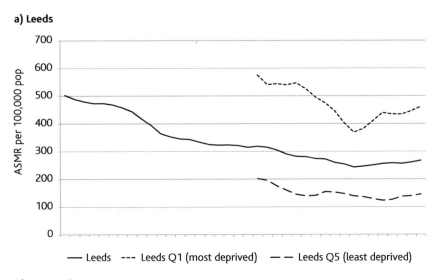

—— Leeds   --- Leeds Q1 (most deprived)   — — Leeds Q5 (least deprived)

b) Liverpool

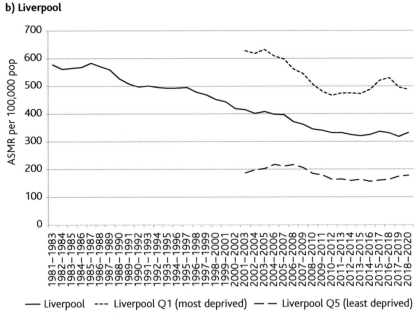

—— Liverpool   --- Liverpool Q1 (most deprived)   — — Liverpool Q5 (least deprived)

Figure 2.4: Age-standardised mortality rates (ASMRs) for males aged 0–64 years, for four English cities and their 20 per cent most and least deprived neighbourhoods, 1981–2019 (continued)

c) Bristol

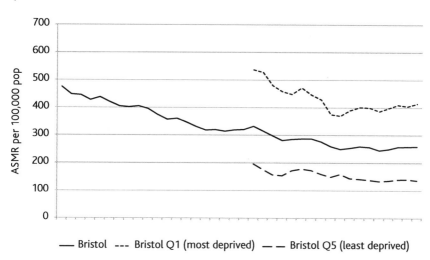

— Bristol   --- Bristol Q1 (most deprived)   — — Bristol Q5 (least deprived)

d) Sheffield

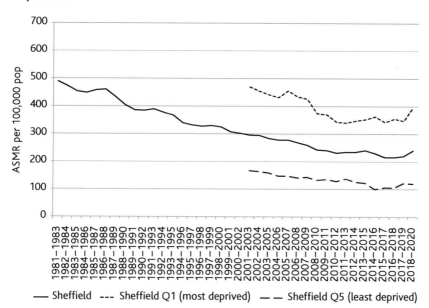

— Sheffield   --- Sheffield Q1 (most deprived)   — — Sheffield Q5 (least deprived)

Notes: Refer to the notes at the end of this book for full description[19]
Source: Calculated from ONS mortality and population data

rates (especially premature mortality rates) have worsened to a greater degree among females[10] – the likely causes of that will be discussed in the next chapter. However, rates for males have obviously also been badly affected, as we have already shown in a number of charts.

With regard to age, Figure 2.5 shows that the rate of improvement either decreased or went into reverse in every single age group. This is taken from published analyses of changes in life expectancy in Scotland between 2000 and 2017.[29] Bars above the horizontal axis indicate improvement in life expectancy; bars below the axis indicate a worsening. The contrast between the earlier (darker bars) and later periods (lighter bars) across all age bands is obvious.

What about causes of death? Taken from the same research paper,[29] Figure 2.6 shows a similar analysis, this time not by age group but for all the specific causes of death. Again, the slower improvement, or in many cases a worsening of rates, in the second period compared to the first is clear for virtually every cause of death. This is an important finding: the fact that adverse changes have been seen for such a broad set of causes is relevant information when it comes to understanding what has been going on. That said, however, Figure 2.6 also shows that some causes of death have been more affected than others: among both males and females, changes in rates of death from heart disease (IHD) and drug-related causes stand out. We explore this further in Chapter 3, where the significance of all the evidence presented here is assessed in detail. Note that the analyses shown in Figures 2.5 and 2.6 are for Scotland. However, similar analyses by age and causes of death for England and Wales have shown similar results.[21,30]

Beyond measures of mortality and life expectancy

Although this book is principally concerned with changes to life expectancy and mortality rates, death is an 'end point'; we also have to understand the 'pathways' and processes that lead to it.[33] Alongside changes to overall death rates in the population, we would therefore also expect to see changes in morbidity (illness) rates – including poor mental health experienced by the population. Recent published evidence for England and Scotland shows precisely this – worsening mental health in the population, particularly among younger and working-age groups. Figure 2.7 shows trends in 'psychological distress'[34] from three national surveys for three broad age groups: the data show increases in rates of poor mental health from the early 2010s onwards for those aged 16–34 and 35–64 years.[35]

It's also possible to combine measures of 'general health' (based on survey questions which ask people to rate how good or bad their health is) with mortality data to provide estimates of not simply how long people are living, but how long they are living *in good health*. This measure – healthy life

Figure 2.5: Contribution of changes in age-specific mortality to the change in life expectancy trends, Scotland, males and females

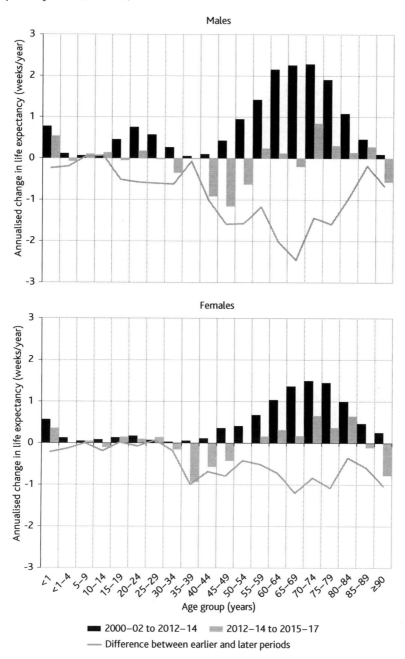

Notes: Refer to the notes at the end of this book for full description.[31]

Source: Ramsay et al 2020[29]

Figure 2.6: Contribution of changes in cause-specific mortality to the change in life expectancy trends, Scotland, males and females

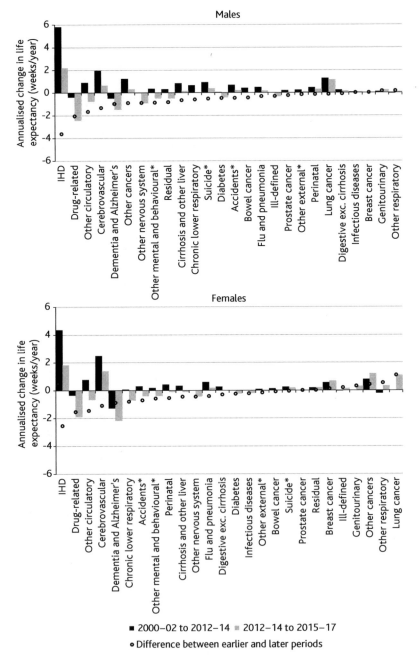

Notes: Refer to the notes at the end of this book for full description.[32]
Source: Ramsay et al 2020[29]

Figure 2.7: Trends in psychological distress in Great Britain (GB), Scotland and England by age, 1991–2019

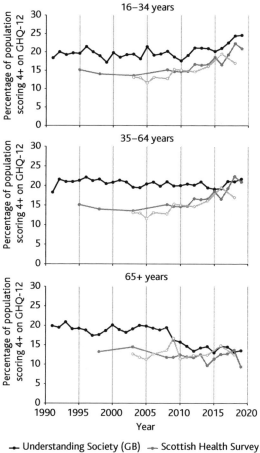

Notes: Refer to the notes at the end of this book for full description.[37]
Source: Zhang et al 2023[35]

expectancy – is arguably a more informative measure than life expectancy alone: there's a big difference between someone dying aged 80 years after six months' poor health, and someone dying at the same age after 10 years' poor health. Recent analyses for Scotland for the years 1995–2019 show quite remarkable changes in this measure in the ten years prior to the pandemic: a decline of two years in the country as a whole, with sharper reductions in the poorest 20 per cent of neighbourhoods – meaning that by 2019 people living in such areas were, on average, living only around 47 years in good health.[36] That's a truly extraordinary statistic in such a wealthy society. These trends are shown in Figure 2.8.

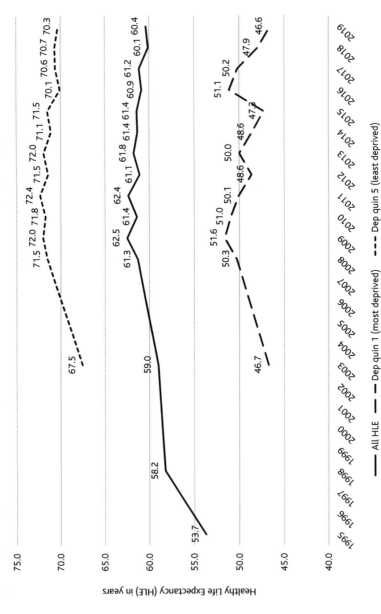

Figure 2.8: Healthy Life expectancy, Scotland and its 20 per cent most and least socioeconomically deprived populations, 1995–2019

Notes: Refer to the notes at the end of this book for full description.[38]
Source: Walsh et al 2022[36]

The impact of COVID-19 on mortality rates

That the COVID-19 pandemic 'exposed existing inequalities' in the UK has become almost a cliché. But, hackneyed statement or not, it's true. As already pointed out, the UK is one of the most unequal high-income countries on the planet – and certainly *the* most unequal in Western Europe.[27] In those circumstances, it's hardly surprising that the arrival of a pandemic would disproportionately affect more disadvantaged groups: this is for a myriad of reasons, including pre-existing poor health (linked to poverty), greater occupational hazards and other vulnerabilities.[39–43] Should we be surprised, therefore, that in England death rates from COVID-19 in 2020–22 were twice as high among those living in the most deprived neighbourhoods as compared to those in the least deprived, and among the Black population compared to the White population?[44] And, as COVID-19 came hard on the heels of a decade of widening mortality inequalities in the UK (as shown in many of the charts in both this and the last chapter), it's hardly surprising that the pandemic further exacerbated an already dire situation: mortality rates among the poorest increased more, inequalities in mortality and life expectancy widened further.

And it seems highly unlikely that things are going to improve any time soon. At the time of writing, the UK is in a cost-of-living crisis. Important modelling work has shown that because of the well-understood links between poverty and poor health, this will likely further increase premature mortality rates in the population.[45,46]

We discuss further these other, additional, impacts on mortality rates in Chapter 6.

What does all this mean for health inequalities in the UK?

It's very clear from the evidence presented so far – increasing death rates in the more deprived areas of the UK contrasting with continuing improvements in less deprived areas – that inequalities in mortality and life expectancy have widened considerably since the early 2010s. It hardly seems necessary to quantify the scale of this; however, as with some of the other analyses shown here, it is nonetheless important to do so. If health inequalities are to be narrowed – and this has been the stated aim of governments in the UK for many decades – then they need to be measured precisely in the first place.

The measurement of health inequalities is a complex topic.[47] They can be measured in both *absolute* terms (crudely, the difference in the rate between socioeconomic groups) or *relative* terms (equally crudely, how many times higher the rate is in one group, compared to the other[48]). The debate that has been played out in journal papers regarding whether one measure is 'better' than the other is not one with which we need to concern ourselves here: what matters is that to fully understand the nature and scale of societal inequality – and changes to that inequality – you need to be aware of what *both* these measures show. However, it is even more important to understand that, as a result of the changes to mortality rates that have taken place in recent years, we are now in a *new era of health inequality* in the UK.

We say that because, prior to these recent changes, absolute inequalities were declining in the UK, while relative inequalities were widening. This is because although the health (mortality) of the whole population was improving, it was doing so to a greater extent among less deprived populations compared to more deprived populations.[49] However, as we have

Figure 2.9: Slope Index of Inequality (SII) and Relative Index of Inequality (RII) for all-cause mortality rates by deprivation quintile, males, Scotland and England, 2001–17

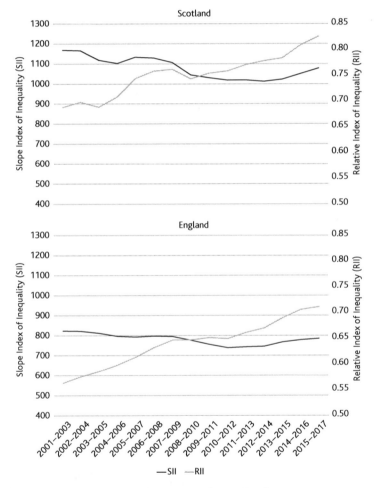

Notes: Refer to the notes at the end of this book for full description.[51]
Source: Walsh et al 2020[20]

shown, since 2012 mortality rates among more deprived populations have gone into reverse – they have not improved, they have become worse. And, as a consequence, we now have increasing absolute *and* relative inequalities. We can see this clearly in Figure 2.9: the SII and the RII are absolute and relative measures of inequalities, respectively.[50]

In this chapter we have presented evidence of the unprecedented changes to life expectancy and mortality rates in the UK, with increasing death rates among poorer populations and the resulting widening of inequalities. We have demonstrated when exactly the changes occurred, quantified their scale and showed how they have affected both sexes, all age groups and all main common causes of death. We have demonstrated how the trends have been exacerbated by the COVID-19 pandemic, and are likely to be made yet worse by the cost-of-living crisis that so many in the country are currently enduring. In the next chapter we use all that evidence alongside yet more to understand the causes of these astonishing changes – changes that have affected so many people, in so many tragic ways, across different parts of the UK.

Frances

One can only wonder how history will judge a government of a wealthy, western, 'developed' nation which, in the early part of the 21st century, decided to financially punish the poorer members of society – if they happened to have an extra bedroom in their house.

It sounds almost comic, like something from Monty Python, or perhaps the Theatre of the Absurd. But this was one of many measures included in the UK Conservative-Liberal Democrat coalition government's Welfare Reform Act of 2012.[1] And for the hundreds of thousands of people affected, it was (and still is) anything but funny.

The legislation meant that people who lived in public housing ('social housing', or what used to be called 'council housing') lost housing benefit if they had any 'spare' bedrooms: a 14 per cent reduction for one extra room, a 25 per cent reduction for two. On average this meant that people who were already on an extremely low income were losing between £50 and £100 per month.[2-5] In most areas of the country, the general lack of social housing meant that very few people were able to move to smaller, more affordable accommodation to escape this financial penalty.[6-9]

The impact of what has been commonly referred to as the 'bedroom tax'[10] has – as just one component of the much larger package of 'welfare reform' measures introduced since 2010 – been considerable. The UK government's own evaluation published in 2015 showed that it had resulted in greater levels of poverty and debt, with over three-quarters of those affected having to cut back on buying basics such as food.[11] Independent research undertaken in the north of England showed that it had 'increased poverty and had broad-ranging adverse effects on health, well-being and social relationships'.[2] In other words, it had created severe hardship.

Some of the more extreme stories of hardship made it into the press. The year after the measure came into force, the *Liverpool Echo* reported the case of Elaine Jones, a young mother whose crime was to have three bedrooms when only she and her son lived at home.[12] With mounting debts resulting from the loss of housing benefit, and unable to cope, she swallowed 29 sleeping tablets, but somehow survived. The case of 53-year-old Stephanie Bottrell received national media attention. Fearing either further financial stress or having to move house because of the bedroom tax, Stephanie climbed a motorway safety barrier and walked into the path of a lorry. Her suicide note blamed the government for her death.[13,14]

The reason that Frances McCormack had a spare bedroom was particularly tragic. Its previous occupant, her beloved son, Jack, had killed himself in 2013 when only 16 years old. However, Frances, a school cook in a small town in Yorkshire in England, was described as a strong person who, two years after Jack's death, was trying to move on and deal with her grief: she had started going out more, and was keeping herself busy with a range of activities including going to the gym and even contributing to the local council's suicide prevention programme. To her friend, whose partner had recently passed away and who had been supported by Frances through her own difficult time, she had been 'my rock'.[15]

However, as a school cook, Frances was on a low income and the imposition of the bedroom tax had led to severe financial difficulties. She had actually penned a letter to the Prime Minister, David Cameron, highlighting the unfairness of her situation and the tax in general. On 9 August 2015 she was served an eviction notice for the house in which she had lived for many years, and in which she had brought up her children. The following day Frances killed herself. The eviction notice and the undelivered hand-written letter to the Prime Minister were found nearby.[15]

One can only wonder how history will judge a government of a wealthy, western, 'developed' nation which, in the early part of the 21st century, rather than help its desperate people in times of need, instead pushed them to – and over – the edge.

Why have mortality rates and life expectancy changed in the UK?

A war without bullets.
Cathy McCormack, 'The Wee Yellow Butterfly'[1]

The changes to life expectancy and mortality rates that have taken place in the UK since the early 2010s have been nothing short of extraordinary. More than that, they have been tragic. Why has this happened?

The numbers involved, and the horrific stories of those affected, mean we need to be absolutely clear about the causes. With that in mind, in 2021 and 2022 we undertook a large-scale exercise in which we systematically assessed all the available evidence for what has happened: what it showed, how strong or weak it was, how plausible it was, how it tallied with other evidence regarding what affects the health of populations, and lots more.[2] And the answer – published in May 2022 and since echoed by yet more research findings that have emerged in the intervening period – was very clear: what's happened is best explained by the economic policies introduced by the UK government since 2010. Or to be more succinct: it's about austerity.

What is austerity?

Austerity is effectively about cuts to government spending. That's not how an economist would ever define it – in fact, they would be deeply unhappy with such a definition. They would use much more complex terms such as 'fiscal consolidation', 'government deficit reduction', 'automatic stabilisers' and many others that mean a lot to economists but not necessarily much to other people. We'll look at those more complicated definitions in the next chapter when we compare the experiences of different countries: for such international analyses, comparable and tightly defined economic definitions of austerity are very important.

In much simpler terms, austerity in the UK has very much been about cuts to government (public) spending. As we mentioned in the opening chapter, it was introduced in 2010 by the coalition government led by David Cameron and Nick Clegg, with George Osborne in charge of financial affairs as Chancellor. On being elected to power in the period following the recession of 2008/09, the new government's stated aim was to achieve economic growth by reducing the gap between government spending and income from taxes, in order to reduce the national debt that had accumulated during the financial crisis and the bailout of the banks (all formulated into the slogan, 'cut the deficit').[3,4] The extent to which these policies were more about ideology (reducing the role of the state in society is a key Conservative Party 'value'[5]) than an effective means of improving the economy has been discussed at length by others,[6] not least because UK economic growth in the subsequent period was slower than in other countries facing similar post-recession challenges.[7–9] However, this is not the focus of our analysis here; rather, our focus is to understand how these policies – irrespective of their motivation or economic effectiveness – have had such an adverse impact on the health of the UK population.

The components of austerity in the UK: what, where and how much?

The cuts to UK government spending have been on a truly mammoth scale. It's hard to be absolutely sure of the precise figure because estimates vary. However, recent analyses suggest that by 2019 annual spending was down by around £91 billion as compared to pre-austerity levels.[10] To put that in context, that's more than the gross domestic product (GDP) of entire countries like Croatia, Bulgaria and even Oman.[11] Over the period 2010–19, the cuts add up to a total reduction of approximately £540 billion. These are changes on an extraordinary level.

Although most UK government departments were affected, the two biggest areas of budget reduction were local government funding (impacting, therefore, on the provision of local public services) and social security.

Looking first at cuts to local government funding, it's hard to overemphasise their significance. The services provided by local councils across the land are vital to a basic functioning of civilised society. Education, housing, public health,[12] environmental services, libraries, other cultural services such as museums and, of course, a broad range of social services are all provided by local government to their population. As we saw a glimpse of in the story of Rachel (and as we shall see later in Paul's story), those social services are of paramount importance to those living in more challenging circumstances. They include adult and elderly social care, child protection, homelessness services, alcohol and drugs services, some aspects of mental health, criminal justice, welfare rights, assistance for carers, and so much more.[13]

However, all these services are the very ones affected by the policies of austerity. Between 2010 and 2016, funding for the local government section of (what was then called[14]) the Department for Communities and Local Government was more than halved:[15] once this reduction was passed on to individual local authorities, their ability to maintain all these vital services was significantly compromised. It limited the amount they could *spend*.[16]

Reductions in levels of council spending in the following years varied considerably across the UK. Detailed analyses by Mia Gray and Anna Barford at Cambridge University showed that – on average – English authorities were worse affected than those in Scotland and Wales.[17] This was because, while the cuts to English local government were administered directly from Westminster, in Scotland and Wales they were filtered through the devolved governments via reductions in the block grants, and the Scottish and Welsh governments were thereby able to partially mitigate their effects.[16] Thus, between 2009/10 and 2016/17, average reductions in council spending were 24 per cent across local authorities in England, but 11.5 per cent and 12 per cent in Scotland and Wales, respectively. However, within each nation, the scale of spending cuts also varied to a considerable degree. For example, while Scotland may have been less affected than England overall, spending in Glasgow, its largest city, was cut by 29 per cent, contrasting with neighbouring East Renfrewshire, where council spending actually *increased* by around 2 per cent in the same period. Similarly in Wales, reductions were notably higher in Denbighshire (23 per cent) than in the likes of Powys (7 per cent). However, in England both the overall level of spending reduction and the variation across areas were on a much greater scale. Gray and Barford showed that, of around 200 British local authority areas analysed, almost one quarter experienced spending cuts of 30 per cent or more, and they were all situated in England. Across England, cuts ranged from around 45 per cent in places like Salford and South Tyneside in the north, to around 5 per cent in Hampshire and Surrey in the south.[16]

That contrast between Salford and South Tyneside, on the one hand, and Hampshire and Surrey, on the other, is not coincidental. And what connects those places in the north of England with Glasgow in Scotland and Denbighshire in Wales is that they are all among the most socioeconomically deprived local authority areas in their respective countries. This is a key feature of how austerity has been implemented in the UK: the worst-affected areas are generally those that were already much poorer to start with. This is true of local government funding – but even more so of social security cuts.

Social security has been defined as the 'protection that a society provides to individuals and households to … guarantee income security, particularly in cases of old age, unemployment, sickness, invalidity, work injury, maternity or loss of a breadwinner'.[18] In other words – and as it has been described elsewhere in this book – it is a social 'safety net': something we should all be able to rely on to help us in times of need.

However, that net has been pulled apart. Like the reduction in local government funding, the scale of the cuts to social security in the UK has been breathtaking. As originally planned in 2010, £47 billion was to be cut from the annual budget by 2021.[19] As with the overall austerity figure, estimates of the total savings achieved by that point vary, and it seems likely that the final figure achieved may well have been less. Nonetheless, all estimates equate to cuts of tens of billions of pounds.[20–25] Again, to put those figures in the same kind of context as before, £47 billion equates to more than the GDP of countries like Jordan or Latvia; even half of it equates to the GDP of Iceland. These are truly enormous amounts of money.

The raft of cuts to social security was carried out in stages. The first set of 'reforms' covered the period 2010–15, implemented by the Coalition Government. These included the changes introduced through the 2012 Welfare Reform Act,[26,27] and others implemented in different government budgets throughout the period. The second set of reforms was implemented from 2015 onwards by the subsequent Conservative government, and included the 2016 Welfare Reform and Work Act.[28]

The full set of reforms is too long to list here (there were around 150 in the first period alone)[29] – others have sought to list them in their entirety.[23,30,31] However, some of the key changes include:

- *A benefit 'freeze'*: from 2016/17, the value of benefits for working-age people was not to increase for four years, meaning a cut in real terms once inflation was taken into account. Prior to that (from 2013), increases were limited to 1 per cent, which again amounted to a cut in the years when inflation was above that level (which it was in three out of the four years[32]). Even before these changes, the method for increasing benefits each year was changed to a lower measure of inflation, resulting in their real value declining over time.[33]
- *Universal Credit*: this replaced, and combined, six separate working-age social security benefits. Its piloting and later expansion was beset with problems and controversy, in particular because of the five- (initially six) week delay before payments are made. This delay was described by a House of Lords inquiry as something which 'entrenches debt, increases extreme poverty and harms vulnerable groups disproportionately'.[34] While 'hardship loans' and advance payments from the Department for Work and Pensions (DWP) could be applied for to help with this delay, the resulting deductions from future payments have been implicated in increased levels of destitution.[35] Introduced first in 2010, changes to Universal Credit implemented in 2016 also meant that payments would start to be withdrawn at lower levels of earnings.
- *Sanctions*: one of the key elements of the 2012 Welfare Reform Act was an increased level of 'conditionality' associated with receipt of social security benefits. This meant that if claimants did not meet particular conditions (such as attending interviews or demonstrating availability for work), their payments would be reduced or stopped. The changes

introduced in 2012 created more conditions for groups such as single parents and employed people on low wages. They also increased the length of time for which sanctions could be in place, and introduced a system of 'escalating sanctions'.[36] The average length of sanctions imposed in 2022 was almost three months:[37] in effect, this can mean people being left for three months without the means to live. While the UK government argued that conditionality and sanctions would encourage people into work, their own analyses (which they were finally forced to release in 2023[38]) showed that the measures were ineffective – people who were sanctioned actually took longer to find work than those who were not.[39,40]

- *Disability-related benefits*: the first set of changes saw the existing Disability Living Allowance replaced by a new benefit called Personal Independence Payment (PIP). Importantly, this was accompanied by much stricter and more frequent medical assessments of the type in the story of Michael O'Sullivan. Similarly, Incapacity Benefit and related payments for people with disabilities and/or health issues were replaced by Employment and Support Allowance (ESA) – again introduced alongside stricter medical tests and with more 'conditionality' attached. From 2016 the level of ESA given to eligible new claimants was also reduced.

- *Child benefit*: changes included a three-year freeze in the value of payments from 2011/12, again resulting in a cut in real terms.

- *Housing benefit*: a number of changes were implemented, including the so-called 'bedroom tax' (highlighted in the story of Frances McCormack) whereby people living in public ('social') housing had their benefit reduced if it was deemed (based on the size of their household) that they had at least one spare bedroom. The policy mainly affected social housing tenants in England: the Scottish Government compensated affected tenants in Scotland with additional money ('discretionary housing payments'), and similar actions were taken in Wales and Northern Ireland.[41–43] In addition, the amount of housing benefit given to private renters was reduced considerably through a series of significant changes to eligibility criteria. This amount remained frozen for many years even though rents increased substantially over the time period.[21,44]

- *Tax credits*: payments and eligibility for both Working Tax Credit and Child Tax Credit (additional benefits for people who were working but still on a low income) were reduced. The second set of changes included limiting the number of eligible children for Child Tax Credit to two (known as the 'two child limit' – see next bullet point).

- *Two child limit*: not only were child tax credits limited to two children, but other benefits, including those provided via Universal Credit, were limited as well. Aside from representing a major cut in income for larger families, these changes achieved notoriety through including a so-called 'rape clause' whereby an exemption was granted for an additional child if the mother could provide proof that the baby was conceived as a result of sexual assault – a demand described by one Member of Parliament as 'one of the most inhumane and barbaric policies ever to emanate from Whitehall'.[45]

- The introduction of a '*benefit cap*', that is, a limit on the total amount of social security payments a workless household can receive. Initially limited to the level of the average weekly wage of an employed person (from 2013), it was then further lowered (in 2016) to a maximum of £20,000 per year (or £23,000 in London). Like the two child limit, this particularly affected larger families, including families with children.

- *Pension credit*: first introduced in the early 2000s to help low-income pensioners, the 'saving credit' component of this benefit (which provided payments for those with a small amounts of savings) was first frozen (in 2011) and then had the eligibility threshold raised (in 2012).[46] Rules were also later (in 2019) changed for 'mixed age' couples (that is, where one is above and one below pension age): this effectively defined both individuals as 'working age' and therefore prevented any claims for Pension credit or pension-age housing benefit being made.[47]

- *Income support and conditionality for lone parents*: lone parents were previously entitled to receive income support without the need to seek work if their youngest child was under 10 years old (that had been reduced from 16 years old by the previous Labour government). This age limit was reduced to seven years old in 2010, to five years old in 2012, and to three years old in 2017.

- Other changes included: the reduction of *Council Tax Support* (as the name suggests, this provided financial help to pay council [local government] tax); yet more reductions in payment levels if any '*non-dependent*' people (for example, elderly relatives or adult children) lived in a claimant's household; *mortgage interest support* being reclassed as a loan; and much more.

The vast number of different cuts (or 'reforms') means that huge numbers of the population have been affected. A precise figure is hard to come by. However, we know that in Great Britain there are around *nine million* low-income households:[48] as these are defined in terms of being in receipt of some sort of benefit or tax credit, then it's a reasonable assumption that the number of people directly affected by these changes is around that number. That's a truly extraordinary figure. These are people whose low level of income means they require help from the state, yet the changes mean that they have received either less help, or no help at all. However, within the spectrum of all those affected, the impact on some groups has been even greater than on others.

Independent analyses have shown that the cuts have been 'regressive': in other words, the very poorest have been affected the very most. Figure 3.1, taken from analyses published by the Equality and Human Rights Commission,[49] shows the estimated change in net household income caused by tax and welfare reforms by 2021/22. In short, the poorest lose about 10 per cent of their (already low) income; the richest lose nothing.

Within that overall regressive picture, lone parents have been particularly affected, as have the disabled members of our population: this is clear from the number of social security reforms that have been directly targeted at them. As members of ethnic minority groups are also more likely to have lower incomes (especially in England[51,52]) – reflecting entrenched inequalities in society generally – they have also been disproportionately affected. Analyses have also shown that the cuts to social security (alongside other aspects of austerity) have had a particular impact on women. This is for a number of reasons. First, women are more likely to be on a low income: this relates to women having more unpaid caring responsibilities, meaning they can work fewer hours and earn less money. Second, as a consequence of being on a lower income, more women than men receive social security payments, and are thus more likely to have been affected by the cuts. Third, many of the groups most affected are either predominantly female (for example, lone parents, single pensioners) or are more likely to have female carers (for example, those with disabilities). On top of all this, women have been more affected by other aspects of austerity: for example, public sector pay freezes and job losses were introduced, and many more women work in the public sector (particularly on a part-time basis); and those greater caring responsibilities also mean that women have not only lost more income, but have also been more affected by the loss of services that provided support to carers.[49,53–60]

Of course, all these population categories – lone parents, ethnic minorities, people with a disability, females, those on the lowest income – overlap (or 'intersect'[61]) to a huge degree, creating the potential for the effects to be exacerbated for people in multiply disadvantaged groups. Analyses aimed at quantifying the financial loss of the social security cuts showed that: low-income women lost considerably more than low-income men; women aged 35–44 years (an age band which includes many lone parents) lost around four times more than males the same age; and the poorest single parents (the vast majority of whom are women) were estimated to have lost as much as 25 per cent of their total income.[49] Similarly, while it was estimated that White women on a low income had lost 11 per cent of their annual income, as compared to 8 per cent for equivalently poor White men, the equivalent figures for the Asian population were 19 per cent and 10 per cent, respectively.[55]

A series of detailed geographical analyses by Christina Beattie and Steve Fothergill at Sheffield Hallam University mapped the parts of the UK most

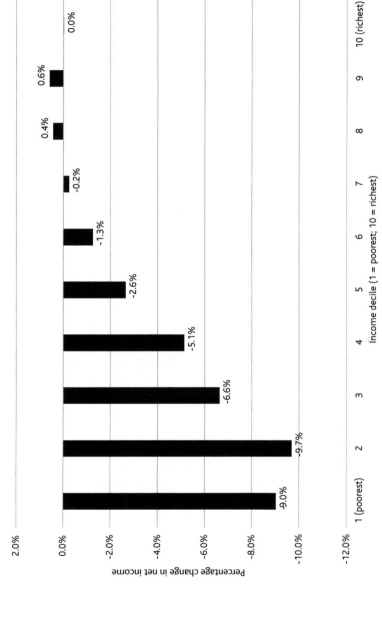

Figure 3.1: Percentage impact of tax and welfare reforms by household net income decile, 2021–22 tax year, Great Britain

Notes: Refer to the notes at the end of this book for full description.[50]
Source: Portes and Reed 2018[49]

affected by these remarkable changes to the social security system.[22,23] As with cuts to local government funding, the most deprived areas have suffered the most: this is hardly surprising, as cuts that are targeted at the poorest members of society will impact more in areas where more poorer people live. Thus, areas that have lost their former industries (for example, former mining or steel towns), seaside towns well past their glory days and particularly deprived London boroughs were all highlighted in the analyses; as in the case of council spending cuts, this contrasted greatly with the experience of wealthier areas in southern England. According to the authors, a 'key effect' of the reforms has been the resulting 'widening of the gap in prosperity' across the country. Echoing the work of others, those most affected were shown to include families with children (particularly lone-parent families), ethnic minority groups and also social housing tenants of working age.

In combination, the scale of cuts, both to vital local services and to the incomes of the poorest and most vulnerable in society via reductions in social security payments, has been astonishing. But how have these cuts resulted in the changes to mortality and life expectancy trends that were presented in the last two chapters? In other words, how does austerity impact on health?

How does austerity impact on health?

To answer this question, we have to understand first of all what causes good and bad health in any population, and what the so-called 'causal pathways' (the processes that lead to good or bad health) are. Key to this is understanding the importance of income and poverty, alongside the many other so-called 'social determinants' of health.

The evidence (1): austerity and poverty

There is a mass of international evidence, arguably going back centuries rather than just decades, of the relationship between income and health. Generally speaking, better income equates to better health, and within that income-and-health spectrum, poverty is very bad for you.[62-66] Put more bluntly, poverty kills. And austerity has increased poverty levels in the UK.

Increased poverty in the UK

The evidence for this comes from multiple sources. First, looking at routine statistical monitoring, Figure 3.2 shows trends in 'relative poverty' both for children and for the whole population pre and post implementation of austerity policies; relative poverty is the measure of poverty that is recommended by independent organisations like the Joseph Rowntree Foundation.[67,68] We have already seen that families with children have

Figure 3.2: Trends in relative poverty (after housing costs), UK, 2005–20, children and total population

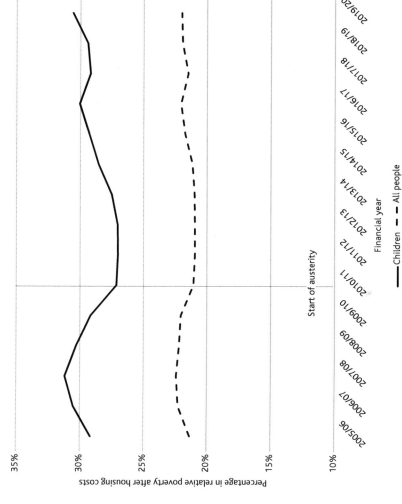

Source: Joseph Rowntree Foundation (calculated from DWP Households Below Average Income dataset)[68]

been particularly affected by the social security cuts, and the trends in child poverty show a marked increase in the ten years following the start of austerity policies. Overall levels of relative poverty have also increased, although not to the same extent. More detailed analyses of the same data show notable increases in poverty rates among pensioners and working-age adults with children.[68]

These trends tell a clear story. However, evidence also comes from studies which examined the relationship between austerity and particular facets of poverty.

Writing today, it seems hard to imagine a time when food banks were not an integral part of UK society. We see them featured regularly in newspapers and on our television screens; they appear in TV soap operas; and food bank donation areas are prominently displayed in our supermarkets. Indeed, for many people, buying extra items for those collections has become a regular part of their weekly shopping trip. Yet, prior to 2010, they *hardly existed*. In the words of researchers at Glasgow and Heriot-Watt universities, they were a 'very marginal phenomenon'. The researchers reported that in 2010/11 the Trussell Trust – the largest food bank provider in the UK – only had 35 food banks across all of England; by 2019/20 they had almost 1,300 (from which almost two million food parcels were distributed). That's an increase of around 3,600 per cent – a truly extraordinary change. Figure 3.3 shows those very figures – the number of food parcels distributed every year by the Trussell Trust between 2010/11 and 2019/20. In detailed statistical analyses, the Glasgow and Heriot-Watt authors showed that particular aspects of the UK government's 'welfare reform' programme had driven this dramatic increase: the low value of social security payments themselves, the roll-out of Universal Credit, sanctions and the bedroom tax were all highlighted.[69]

Other research showed similar results in terms of who was forced to use food banks: when surveyed back in 2016, around two-thirds of users were dependent on social security benefits, and about half cited low income and changes or delays to benefits as the main reason for their referral.[72,73] Further detailed evidence of the clear link between the introduction of austerity and increased food bank use has since emerged, including a 'systematic review'[74] published in 2021.[75]

The UK government themselves recently estimated that, astonishingly, more than two million people in the UK were forced to use food banks in 2021/22.[76] However, analyses by the Trussell Trust have shown that this is just the tip of the iceberg: in the same twelve-month period, over *eleven million* people in the UK experienced 'food insecurity'[77,78] – in other words, they went hungry. Eleven million people! Austerity policies have fundamentally changed the society in which people in the UK now live.

Similarly, levels of homelessness have increased across many parts of the UK in recent times. Analyses for England undertaken in the early years

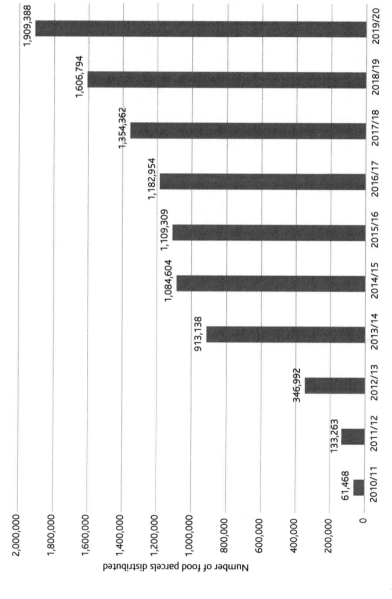

Figure 3.3: Numbers of parcels distributed by food banks in the Trussell Trust network, 2010/11 to 2019/20

Notes: Refer to the notes at the end of this book for full description.[71]
Source: Trussell Trust[70]

of austerity demonstrated a clear relationship between increased rates of homelessness and cuts to social security benefits.[79] Since then, multiple commentators, analysts and even (presumably in a careless, 'off-message', moment) a UK government minister have highlighted austerity's impact on increased levels of homelessness, including the numbers forced to sleep 'rough' on our streets.[80–83]

(Although perhaps the Government minister's admission – made in 2018 – was not a big surprise: seven years earlier, a leaked letter to the Prime Minister from the office of another prominent cabinet minister suggested that the process of 'welfare reform' risked making 40,000 families in the UK homeless.)[84]

On a number of measures, therefore, austerity has been shown to have increased poverty across UK society. And the consequences of this for the health of those affected are very clear.

Poverty and health

Poverty damages your health in lots of different, and quite complex, ways. First, and perhaps most obviously, being poor means you can't afford to buy the *material goods and services* that are needed to keep you healthy, and which – more broadly – allow you to participate fully in society. Things like being able to afford to live in a decent home, and being able to afford to pay the rent and bills to stay in your home and keep it warm. Also, having the money to travel to important places: health service appointments, job interviews or just to meet up with friends and family and so avoid becoming socially isolated. And, of course, being able to not just eat, and avoid hunger and the need for those food banks discussed earlier, but to eat *healthily*. In the UK healthy food tends to be more expensive, while the cheaper options are more unhealthy, processed foods: recent research by The Food Foundation has shown that it would cost poorer families in the UK almost 75 per cent of their disposable income to follow UK government healthy eating guidance.[85]

Second, being unable to do these things, worrying about paying bills and whether or not you can put afford to put food on your kids' dinner plates at night, all causes enormous levels of *stress*. And there is very solid biological evidence that stress causes ill-health. Stress, including the type of economic stressors we are discussing here, are very well understood risk factors for a range of chronic health conditions.[86,87] Poverty causes stress, and stress causes physical illness.

Third, these same stressors damage people's *mental health*: being unable to afford life's necessities, and having to deal with many other poverty-related issues like stigma, discrimination, fear, the feeling of being excluded from society, all take their mental toll. There is a huge amount of evidence for this in the international research literature.[88] And aside from everything else associated with that, there is clear evidence that poor mental health can lead to poor physical health. This has been demonstrated in studies for overall ('all-cause') mortality, for deaths from cardiovascular disease and for different types of cancer. For example, after taking into account differences in income, background, previous health conditions, health behaviours (such as, smoking, drinking) and more, people in Britain with high levels of anxiety and depression have been shown to have around 30 per cent higher risk of dying from any cancer (and are up to four times more likely to die from particular types of cancer) and to be around twice as likely to die younger than people with no, or lower levels of, poor mental health.[89,90] The biological processes involved overlap with those through which poverty causes physical ill-health.[86,87]

Fourth, people often deal with the misery of poverty in ways that damage their health – so-called '*coping mechanisms*': these can range from comfort eating and smoking through to excessive alcohol and problematic drug use. Across the UK – indeed, across the world – deaths from these more coping-related conditions (lung cancer [linked to smoking], obesity, alcohol and drug-related causes) are many times more common among the poor than among the rich.[62–64] And then there are what we might call '*non-coping*' *mechanisms* like suicide: in England in 2019, suicide rates were twice as high in more, as compared to less, deprived areas.[91]

In a nutshell, therefore, poverty harms health. If poverty increases, so do deaths: the impact of stress, how people respond to such stressful circumstances, the inability of afford health-protecting factors (a warm house, good food) all combine to take a damaging toll: people die younger, and so death rates go up. *And to a considerable degree, therefore, increases in mortality rates in particular parts of the UK can be very easily understood in terms of the corresponding increases in poverty caused by austerity.*

The evidence (2): austerity and other health 'determinants'

As supremely important as they are, poverty and income are not the only influences on people's health. They interact with many other so-called 'social determinants': these are the multiple, interconnected, societal, economic and environmental conditions that affect everyone's health and well-being, wherever they are. These include housing, employment, the wider environment you live and work in, education, social networks and lots more beside.[62,64,92,93] In public health textbooks, they are presented in an almost bewildering array of diagrams ('models') of differing levels of complexity.[94–96] But, at its heart, this is pretty simple stuff: having money in your pocket; being able to live in a decent, warm house; having a good, rewarding job; having support from friends or others in the community; living in a nice area; being able to access (and afford) decent food – all these things are good for you and your health. Conversely, not being able to have or do these things is not good for you. This represents centuries of public health evidence – but it's also common sense.

Alongside this, health and social care services are also hugely important for everyone: these are the services we all rely on at certain times of our lives – when we are in need, and often when we are at our most vulnerable.

Importantly, the evidence shows that all of these factors that shape people's health have been affected by the policies of austerity. As we have seen from Gray and Barford's analyses – and as was illustrated in Rachel's story – austerity has drastically cut the important services that many people rely on.[16] This includes services like social care, but also others such as those provided by local housing departments which directly impact on the conditions in which people live, and the amenities they are able to access: those 'social determinants' of health. The cuts have been greatest in the poorer areas where we have seen the worst changes to mortality and life expectancy. In that and other ways, therefore, the two key components of austerity – loss of income through cuts to social security and loss of services through cuts to funding – have combined to have an appalling impact on the health of the population. Let's look now at the specific research evidence of the link between these two components of austerity and different aspects of health.

The evidence (3): austerity, illness and death

Poor mental health

We look first at the evidence around mental health: as already mentioned, it's important to understand the 'causal pathways' through which austerity impacts on mortality rates, and poor mental health lies on that pathway, being affected by the same 'stressors' and known to influence poor physical health.

Overall trends in one measure of poor mental health (psychological distress) were shown for all Great Britain in the previous chapter, and a similar worsening of a range of mental health problems has been recorded in various parts of the country;[97,98] however, a considerable number of studies have gone further than just examining trends and have instead analysed in detail the *relationship* between different aspects of mental health and the two main components of austerity. All point to the same damning conclusion regarding austerity's detrimental effect. Examples include:

- a UK-wide study from Oxford University which showed increased levels of depression among people whose housing benefit was reduced;[99]
- analyses from some of the same authors at Oxford which demonstrated notably higher levels of anxiety and depression among those subjected to the benefit cap;[100]

- a study by researchers in Canada that showed worsening mental health among UK housing benefit recipients affected by the bedroom tax;[101]
- Edinburgh University research which showed an association between cuts to social security and prescriptions for anti-depressant medication;[102]
- analyses from the University of Liverpool showing poorer mental health resulting from the introduction of Universal Credit across Britain;[103]
- a study by other researchers in Liverpool which highlighted the relationship between poor mental health and cuts to particular local government services in England;[104]
- research from colleagues at Glasgow University showing poorer mental health among lone parents resulting from the 'conditionality' element for the receipt of benefits;[105]
- further research from the University of Liverpool that demonstrated the relationship between the increased numbers of disabled people having their 'work capability' reassessed (like Michael O'Sullivan) and increased incidence of mental health problems, anti-depressant prescribing and suicides.[106]

These studies have been published in the context of recent international evidence that policies which increase social security generosity and eligibility can protect mental health, while cuts damage it.[107]

Other diseases and mortality/life expectancy

In the previous chapter, we showed that changes to mortality had been seen for virtually all age groups and causes of death. This is reflected in the many studies that have specifically examined the role of austerity in the changing death rates. For overall mortality and life expectancy, this large body of research includes:

- analyses from Public Health Scotland[108] which showed reductions in male and female life expectancy caused by the loss of income due to different 'welfare reforms' (with the worst effects being observed in more deprived areas);[109]
- our own analyses which demonstrated that similar reductions in life expectancy were associated with social security cuts across all local authority areas in Scotland, England and Wales;[110]
- research from the University of York showing cuts to social care, healthcare and public health funding in England accounted for a 'most conservative' estimate of almost 60,000 extra deaths in the first 4–5 years of austerity;[111,112]
- work by researchers at Liverpool University which showed an association between all cuts to local government funding in England and reductions

in life expectancy for males and females – this was true for people of all ages, but also the elderly;[113]

- other analyses led by Kings College London and Oxford University of the effect of austerity on older populations in England which showed increased death rates among those aged 60+ and 85+ years, respectively: these were related to cuts to health and social care budgets, and the loss of social security among those on low incomes.[46,114]

The University of York study included the impact of cuts to healthcare (as well as to social care and public health), and it is worth pointing out here that while National Health Service funding increased in absolute terms in the austerity period, a number of analyses have shown that it did not do so at a level required to deal with societal demands: an ageing population, increased levels of illness and, indeed, the effects of austerity. In essence, funding trends were flat, when they needed to be rising steeply.[115–117]

Analyses of specific illnesses and causes of death include a University of Manchester-led study which showed the link between cuts in local government funding in England and levels of 'multimorbidity' (in other words, people suffering from more than one health condition), and similar analyses from researchers in London demonstrating an association between funding cuts and increased hospital admissions from nutritional anaemia (a marker of malnutrition), especially in more deprived areas.[118,119] Reflecting the earlier discussion of 'coping mechanisms', other studies have examined the impact of austerity (in terms both of funding cuts and of social security cuts) on alcohol- and drugs-related harm. These latter studies include:

- research by the University of Sheffield showing significant reductions in access to addictions services resulting from cuts to funding in England;[120,121]
- a London School of Economics-led study demonstrating the relationship between cuts to local government social care and housing funding and hospital admissions for drugs use;[122]
- a separate study from Liverpool University showing the relationship between cuts to local housing services and drug-related deaths;[123,124]
- and a Great Britain-wide analysis of the relationship between social security cuts and increased drug-related mortality.[125]

It is also worth reflecting on the evidence discussed earlier in this chapter that women on low incomes may have been affected to a greater degree than men by the changes to social security and loss of local services. Has this been reflected in the results of research published to date? Many studies have not actually analysed data for men and women separately; however, of those which did, while results were mixed, several showed worse outcomes for women. This included our own analyses of death rates (shown in Figure 2.3

in the previous chapter), which showed that rates in the poorer areas of Scotland and England had worsened to a greater degree among females, as compared to males.[126] Similarly, particularly adverse trends in life expectancy for women in low-income neighbourhoods were highlighted in separate studies for both England (by researchers at Imperial College London)[127,128] and Wales (by researchers at Cardiff and other universities).[129] In addition, some studies have shown worse *mental health* impacts on females, as compared to males, resulting from austerity policies.[130,131] All that said, as we showed in the first two chapters, we have seen astonishing changes to mortality rates for those living in the 20 per cent most deprived areas right *across the UK*, more or less irrespective of age and gender. And this is explained by the sheer scale of the austerity cuts which have affected all vulnerable populations in the country.

The evidence (4): austerity and child health

Another area in which a considerable amount of research evidence is emerging is in relation to austerity and child health.

We have already shown that the policies of austerity have particularly affected families with children, and that child poverty levels in the UK have increased markedly since those policies were introduced. This chimes with the results of a systematic review of the international evidence showing that austerity policies are linked with higher child poverty (as well as wider 'material deprivation') and also with more babies born with a low birthweight.[132] Being born with a low birthweight is important because it is associated with a higher risk of experiencing a number of health issues later in life.[133–137] And what links austerity to low birthweight is poverty-related stress. There is a considerable evidence base for the adverse impact of stress – including economic 'stressors' (for example, loss of income, poverty) – on birth 'outcomes' such as whether a baby is carried to full term, whether he/she is born underweight and whether the pregnancy miscarries.[136–138] Given this evidence, with colleagues we recently examined trends in the numbers of low birthweight babies and premature births in Scotland. This showed that, following the introduction of austerity, rates of both increased markedly among mothers living in poorer neighbourhoods (Figure 3.4). The results were confirmed by different sets of modelling analyses undertaken to ensure they were not chance findings.

Other analyses of austerity and child health were undertaken by colleagues at Liverpool University, who showed that austerity-implemented cuts to children's centres (these are local authority-run 'Sure Start' centres which provide a range of help to young children and their mothers[141]) were associated with increased levels of childhood obesity.[142] Increased obesity levels resulting

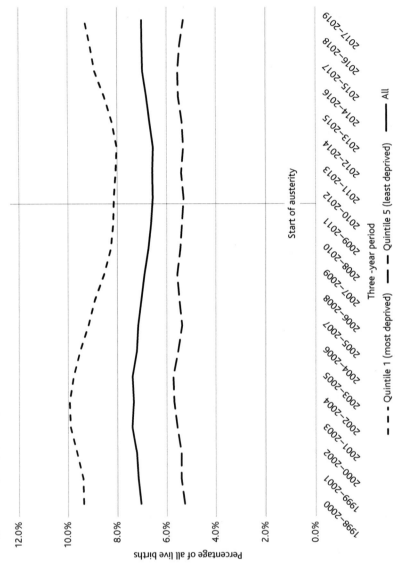

Figure 3.4: Low birthweight babies (as a percentage of all live births), three-year rolling averages, Scotland, 1998–2019

Notes: Refer to the notes at the end of this book for full description.[140]
Source: Watson et al, forthcoming[139]

from the cuts were explained in terms of both *direct* effects (such as from the loss of programmes and services which were specifically aimed at preventing child obesity, such as nutrition advice and programmes promoting healthy child weight) and *indirect* effects (for example, from loss of childcare and social support, and knock-on effects in terms of loss of employment and so on).

Childhood poverty, low birthweight, premature birth and child obesity are all related to a range of problems later in life.[133,143-145] In this way, the effects of austerity in the UK are likely to be with us for many, many years.

The evidence (5): 'qualitative' studies of the impact of austerity on health

As we reflect further at the end of this chapter, in presenting all the evidence of austerity's impact, we have thus far limited ourselves to what are referred to as 'quantitative' studies – that is, those which have statistically *quantified* the association between austerity and health. However, it is also important not to ignore the non-statistical, 'qualitative', accounts of *how* people have been affected by the changes that have been implemented. That is why we share the stories of Michael, Rachel, Frances and others throughout this book. However, a much larger qualitative evidence base of the impacts of austerity has been created through interviews and discussions with those affected. This is a different form of evidence, one in which we can directly hear the voices of those impacted.

As a first example, collaborative research across UK universities has documented the ways in which the introduction of Universal Credit – as a newly introduced benefit with 5–6-week payment delays and the threat of punitive 'sanctions' built into it – has damaged individuals' mental health through the sheer stress of trying to navigate a barely navigable system, and as a result of all the debts (rent arrears, unpaid bills, personal debt) that the payment delays cause.[146,147] Quotes like these from three different Universal Credit claimants in the north-east of England (recorded in 2017) are very typical:

> When you feel like, I can't feed myself, I can't pay my electric bill, I can't pay my rent, well, all you can feel is the world collapsing around you. It does a lot of damage, physically and mentally ... there were points where I did think about ending my life.

> It's not right. I shouldn't have to go to my daughter's and depend on her for something to eat. It should be the other way round. ... It makes you feel so low, especially when you've got to go to the food banks. I don't want to be like this for the rest of my life.

> It's like insidious brutality, this Universal Credit thing.[146]

Other qualitative studies provide us with important insights into the effects of different facets of austerity on the lives – and, importantly, health – of individuals. One study in the south-east of England, for example, focused on the impact of the loss of social care services (brought about by cuts to funding) in the local community.[148] One resident described how the loss of mental health support for her teenage daughter impacted on her own health: 'Some days I have such a bad headache and I'm puking up with the stress because I'm thinking where do I take her, what do I do with her? So, my health suffers because I've nowhere to go [for help].'[148]

Another study, in York, captured the inability of people on reduced social security benefits to eat healthily (something that the Food Foundation's study – which we referred to earlier in the chapter – has also highlighted): 'The reality is that on Universal Credit I cannot provide the recommended amount of fresh fruit and vegetables per day for my children, and I go without more times than not so they can have my share.'[149]

Other studies of poverty and hunger (often termed 'food insecurity' in the research world, as we said earlier) have highlighted not only such lack of nutrition but also people's inability to actually *cook* food because they simply cannot afford to pay fuel bills.[150] Study participants have also articulated the shame they feel at having to rely on the charity of food banks to survive. As one interviewee in the north-east of Scotland put it: 'It's a very humbling experience, very embarrassing and you feel ashamed, but you're desperate.'[150]

Such humiliation and shame are but two of the many emotions that emerge as themes across different qualitative studies – emotions which obviously increase stress levels and ultimately damage health. Indeed, researchers have even created a set of so-called 'austerity ailments' to capture the ways in which austerity impacts on mental health in particular.[151] Alongside humiliation and shame, the other key components are fear and distrust, instability and insecurity, isolation and loneliness, and feeling trapped and powerless. There is clear evidence linking each of these to psychological distress and poor mental health,[151] and they have all been highlighted in different studies. For example, tales of financial *insecurity and instability* abound, such as those voiced earlier by the Universal Credit claimants in north-east England – but there are many, many more. *Fear* (of poverty, and of what the future holds more generally) is a clearly related emotion, as – for example – articulated by participants in another study in the north of England:[152]

> Some days I just sit and I'm crying over absolutely nothing. And the postie [postman] comes and I see a brown envelope and I don't want to open it, because it's either the housing or the benefit, and it's just like, since all the changing over of the different benefits over the last couple of years, that's been the worst time for me, these last two and a half years to three years, benefit-wise.

There's the stress of always worrying are they going to pay me this week? Am I going to be able to pay my bills? Of course in the meantime your rent goes into arrears, your council tax goes into arrears, it has a chain effect. It's relentless ... you go to bed thinking about it and you wake up thinking about it.[152]

As we have discussed, people adopt different 'coping mechanisms' to deal with such fear and stress, many of which are likely to further damage health. For example, this was the only way that one participant in the same study could deal with the stress:

I just used to put meself [myself] in bed, and sleep. I could sleep for days. I knew, if I'm asleep, I don't have to deal with reality, with what's going on. So I would just sleep and sleep. I would wake up and go to the toilet and get a drink of water and just go back to bed. I would lose literally a stone doing that.[152]

Isolation and loneliness is another of these key themes. There are different facets of this: from literally isolating yourself from reality by taking to bed (in the case just cited), to loneliness imposed on vulnerable, elderly people from the loss of their 'Meals on Wheels' service (as described in a study of the effects of austerity in the east of England),[153] to a much broader sense of being 'cut off' from the rest of society by the impact of austerity-driven poverty that was described by this social security claimant in a study in Glasgow:

It stops you from being part of society, because you can't do what you want to do. ... You can't go out for a night out and not worry about what you are spending. When you are working, you can go out once a month and you can really let loose. You can't do that when you are on benefits. ... So you feel like you've lost a bit of your social ... status.[154]

Obviously these, and the other debilitating factors already described, do not occur independently of one another: they interact and overlap, and ultimately converge to have devastating impacts on the health of all those affected. They lead to despair, desperation and illness, as outlined in the final two quotes included here. The first is from a 40-year-old woman from a (unnamed) UK city who survived a suicide attempt after it all became too much:

I looked at my suicide note afterwards. ... Most of it was about the bank (pause) so anyway, yeah, the [benefits] I get tomorrow will go into the overdraft. I literally – I can't phone them because my phone's been cut off and I just – I cannot face going into the branch. ... I don't know what's going to happen now, I really don't.[155]

The second is from the partner of a Universal Credit claimant:

> He was in and out of hospital with his depression, like self-harming and that. It was just horrible. … He spoke to the psychiatrist in the hospital. He was like, we've got no money, what's the point, I can't go out, can't see people, can't even eat properly.[146]

Is it only about austerity?

In this chapter we have outlined the evidence for why austerity has been the principal cause of the changes to mortality and life expectancy, and sought to explain the processes (causal pathways) involved. As mentioned at the outset, this is based in part on a detailed assessment, published in 2022, of all the evidence that was available at that time.[2]

However, as we discuss in more detail in Chapter 5, as evidence of the changing mortality rates slowly emerged over the course of the 2010s, different (non-austerity) 'explanations' were proposed by a variety of individuals and organisations; indeed, in some quarters they continue to be suggested today. The evidence for and against these alternative theories was also assessed in that 2022 report, and it was important to do so for two reasons. First and foremost, we need a fully evidenced understanding of the causes of the changes so we can (hopefully) try to reverse what has happened and return to 'normal' levels of improving population health in the UK. In addition, however, a small number of the other proposed explanations, while not in any way the main drivers of the changes, are still – to a greater or lesser degree – relevant to the overall story. Their potential contribution, therefore, needs to be understood.

Here we very briefly summarise the evidence relating to six alternative suggested explanations included in the 2022 report. We return to some aspects of this discussion in Chapter 6.

Cardiovascular disease (CVD)

What was suggested?

CVD is a generic term covering diseases of the heart and blood vessels; it therefore includes conditions like angina, coronary (or ischaemic) heart disease, strokes and heart failure. It was suggested that the overall stalling of improvement in life expectancy was driven by a stalling of improvement in deaths from CVD specifically; and that the slowdown in improvement in CVD mortality was driven by less improvement and/or a worsening in well-known risk factors such as smoking, obesity and diabetes, as well as a reduction over time in the gains from medical interventions (that is, fewer new treatments were becoming available to continue previous improvements).

Is there anything in it?

Yes – but only up to a point.

As we showed in the previous chapter,[156] alongside drug-related deaths, the changes in mortality rates in Scotland have been greatest for CVD; they have therefore made the largest contribution to the overall 'stalling'. As a risk factor for CVD, changes in obesity rates are also relevant, as we discuss further later in the Chapter (and in Chapter 6).

However, the argument against this as a comprehensive explanation is simple: if it's all about CVD, why have so many other causes of death – entirely unrelated to CVD – been affected? Something else has to be driving all these changes, not just factors relevant to CVD. For example, looking at the underlying data behind Figure 1.4 (in Chapter 1), which shows the dramatic increase in mortality for women under the age of 65 years in Glasgow, only an extremely small proportion of deaths were due to CVD. The same is true when the analyses are extended to all of Scotland.[157,158] CVD is therefore just one of the disease pathways affected by whatever is driving the changed mortality trends overall (that is, austerity), and not a particularly useful alternative 'explanation'.

While smoking, diabetes and obesity are indeed well-evidenced risk factors for CVD, we also know that poverty and deprivation (and their associated stressors) are, in turn, hugely important risk factors for smoking, diabetes and obesity (as well as an important cause of CVD itself, independent of these issues):[159–161] rates and prevalence of all three are hugely 'socially patterned', that is, affecting poorer people to a much larger extent than wealthy people. Poverty and deprivation are good examples of what has been referred to as 'the causes of the causes'.[64,162,163] Thus, the more likely explanation is that changes to rates of CVD mortality have, like many other conditions, been affected by changes to economic conditions (for example, poverty rates) and broader living conditions brought about by austerity policies.

That said, previous increases in obesity are likely to have increased the risk of CVD mortality (and other causes of death, including cancers) since around 2012, and this is likely to have had much worse effects in more deprived areas. The contribution of increased obesity is discussed briefly later in this section and in more detail in Chapter 6.

Drug-related deaths

What was suggested?

Similar to the CVD theory, the suggestion here was that the overall changes to mortality and life expectancy were driven particularly by increases in one condition: in this case, drug-related deaths. This was specifically hypothesised about the situation in Scotland.

Is there anything in it?

Again, yes – but only to a degree.

Drug-related deaths increased considerably in the period in which the overall mortality and life expectancy changes occurred. And while drug-related deaths are a particularly tragic problem in Scotland – rates are amongst the highest of high-income countries, and those rates increased quite dramatically over the period in question – deaths from this cause also rose notably in England and Wales. Furthermore, drug-related deaths occur at younger ages, and the way summary health measures like life expectancy are calculated means that younger deaths have more impact than deaths at older ages do. What's more, younger deaths also affect the trends in premature mortality – trends that we have again highlighted in earlier chapters, including the dramatic changes to early death rates among females in the more deprived areas of Glasgow (Figure 1.4 in Chapter 1). So, in some senses, this is a plausible theory.

However, there are very important reasons why this is all not 'just' about drugs. First, we have seen changes to mortality rates for all different causes of death: it therefore simply cannot be just about drug deaths.[129,164,165] Second, while drug-related deaths are a particular issue for Scotland, the overall changes to life expectancy and mortality rates that we showed in the first two chapters have been very similar in England and Wales, and Northern Ireland, where rates of drug-related deaths are much lower. On top of that, if you actually exclude drug-related deaths from the analyses of premature all-cause mortality trends, the rates still increase sharply from 2012 onwards (including those shown in Figure 1.4 for Glasgow) – and we showed this in the 2022 report.[2]

And finally – and perhaps most importantly of all – there is very strong evidence that the increases in drug-related deaths are themselves associated with the policies of austerity. In this chapter we have already cited a number of studies showing this very issue: increased rates of death from drug-related causes linked to cuts in particular services (including addiction services) as well to loss of income though cuts to social security.[121,125] With regard to the latter, we also spoke to a senior figure in Addiction Services in Scotland who described the issue in these grim terms: 'if you have a highly vulnerable group of people with addiction issues, and you either reduce their income (though reducing their benefits), or take you take it away completely (through benefit sanctions) then what people do is look for oblivion'. As Figure 3.5 shows, the trends in drug deaths in the poorer parts of Scotland show precisely that: within a year or two of the introduction of austerity, people sought a way out. They looked for oblivion.[166,149]

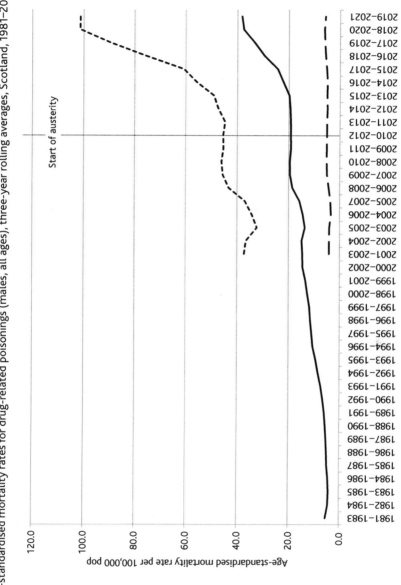

Figure 3.5: Age-standardised mortality rates for drug-related poisonings (males, all ages), three-year rolling averages, Scotland, 1981–2021

Notes: Refer to the notes at the end of this book for full description.[169]
Source: Walsh and McCartney 2023[168]

Deaths from dementia and Alzheimer's disease

What was suggested?

Again, similar to the CVD and drug deaths hypotheses, it was suggested in various quarters that the overall mortality/life expectancy changes had been caused in large part by increased numbers of deaths from one condition: dementia (including, more specifically, Alzheimer's disease).

Is there anything in it?

No. As with drug deaths, the suggestion was based on evidence of really large increases in deaths from this cause over the relevant time period. Analyses also showed that this had not just been caused by the country's ageing population: as we mentioned in Chapter 1, the calculation of the age-standardised mortality rate (as the name suggests) explicitly takes age into account, and this rate for dementia increased by more than 75 per cent between 2002 and 2019.[170] What's more, most of that increase occurred after 2010 – that is, the period in which we are most interested.

The evidence shows[171–173] that this increase has been principally driven by two factors. First, by better detection, and therefore diagnosis, of dementia in primary care (that is, by GPs and others), which in turn led to an increase in dementia being included on death certificates (as certifying doctors were obviously more aware of individuals having the condition); and all of this was probably prompted by national dementia strategies which were put in place in the UK around 15 years ago. Second, it was caused – astonishingly – by changes to the software that is used to apply cause-of-death codes to death certificates. Briefly,[174] this increased the number of times dementia was included on death certificates in particular years – for example, by almost 60 per cent in 2011 in England. In fact, analyses showed that 40 per cent of the increase in recorded deaths from dementia in England between 2001 and 2016 was down to this software glitch.[165,175,176]

Much of this 'increase', therefore, has been artificial; indeed, perhaps contrary to popular perception, the 'age-specific incidence' of dementia in the UK (that is, the number of new cases recorded every year for different age groups) has actually *fallen*, not increased, in recent times.[177,178] On top of all this, the evidence also shows that, in any case, the trend in increased diagnoses pre-dates the overall mortality changes by around a decade. And, as if that weren't enough, the argument against the CVD and drug death hypotheses also applies here: if it were just about deaths from dementia, why have all other causes of death been affected? Finally, dementia mainly affects the elderly: yet the evidence presented in the previous chapter shows changes to death rates at all different age groups. Increasing dementia is therefore a wholly inadequate explanation for the trends.

Deaths from influenza ('flu)

What was suggested?

As we will discuss in further detail in Chapter 5 (in which we deal with the responses of governments and national agencies to the crisis), *'it's just 'flu'* was one of the most frequent 'explanations' given for the changed mortality trends, particularly in the earlier period.

Is there anything in it?

No. It was suggested in those early years because in 2015 (when evidence of the mortality changes was beginning to emerge) there was an increase in the numbers of deaths from influenza.[179,180] Bizarrely, this continued to be the favoured explanation of many organisations for several years[181] – 'bizarrely', because there was so little supporting evidence for its role.[171]

The changes are clearly not due to 'flu for a number of very obvious reasons which are similar to those already discussed in relation to the other theories. First, deaths from 'flu are more common among older populations, but we know that all age groups have been affected. Second, we have seen changes to all causes of death – so it simply cannot just be about deaths from this disease. And third, higher-than-expected mortality has of course been recorded in every year since 2012 – not just in 2015.

Just to hammer home the point, a number of specific analyses have been undertaken to try to quantify the contribution (or otherwise) of influenza to the changed trends, and without exception they have suggested its contribution has been either negligible or nil.[2,171,182] Various complex methods were employed to overcome the problem of under-reporting of influenza deaths: for a variety of reasons, 'flu is not always included as a cause of death on death certificates when it might be potentially relevant. These analyses included trends in deaths from influenza combined with those from pneumonia, broader combinations of ''flu-like illnesses', as well as a study in England which looked at deaths (from any recorded cause) which followed a 'flu-related admission to hospital.[165] None of these analyses found that influenza was likely to be a major contributor to the changed trends. Perhaps a more interesting question, therefore, is why so many people in influential positions continued to argue for this 'explanation'[183] – we return to this in Chapter 5.

Obesity

What was suggested?

Obesity levels increased notably in the UK prior to the mortality changes taking place. As there is good evidence of a causal link between obesity and all-cause mortality (as well as CVD mortality more specifically), it was suggested that the slowdown in improvement in death rates might be explained by the earlier increase in obesity levels in the population.

Is there anything in it?

Yes – but to a relatively small degree.

As we discuss this in more detail in Chapter 6 (when we consider other factors that are important to the recent story of health and health inequalities in the UK), we offer only a brief synopsis here.

In short, we explored this hypothesis for Scotland and England using a data-modelling approach, with the results published in a journal paper in 2022.[184] In this work we sought to quantify the contribution of the earlier increases in obesity to the overall 'stalling' of improvement since 2012. Despite that aim of quantification, for a number of different reasons (relating to the datasets we could use, the quality of the available evidence on the relationship between obesity and mortality, and the assumptions we had to employ), it was virtually impossible to come up with an accurate figure. Importantly, a detailed assessment of possible biases associated with the methods used suggested that the results we did end up with were likely to represent an *overestimate*.

Nonetheless – and with those supremely important caveats in mind – our analyses suggested that between 10 per cent (males) and 14 per cent (females) of the overall 'stalling' of mortality rates in Scotland might be attributable to the earlier increases in obesity; in England, the equivalent figures were notably higher: 20 per cent (males) and 35 per cent (females). To flip those results on their head, however, this means that between 86 per cent and 90 per cent (at least) of the horrific changes to death rates in Scotland, and between 65 per cent and 80 per cent (at least) of the equally appalling changes observed in England, are *not* related to obesity.[185] And so, while we do not ignore obesity (it's a very important issue for public health in the UK and elsewhere, and we will come back to the subject in Chapter 6), it is right that our focus is principally on the effects of austerity policies in causing the mortality and life expectancy changes that we have witnessed in recent years.

Demographic and methodological issues

What was suggested?

A number of different suggestions were made which can probably best (if not very excitingly) be summarised as demographic and methodological issues (stay awake at the back there!). These included the effects of the ageing population, the impact of migration, the suggestion that we had reached the 'natural limit' of life expectancy and even less interesting issues relating to particular datasets and methods used to analyse them.

Is there anything in it?

No, not really. For anyone familiar with studies of population health in the UK, the majority of the suggestions did not really make much sense (which makes it all the more depressing that, as we discuss in Chapter 5, one or two of them were actually cited by UK government ministers who should have known – or at least have been advised – better). Given the lack of supporting evidence for these theories, we mention only a few of them here, and do so only very briefly. For the more committed reader (especially those with a particular interest in specific methodological factors), the full details are included in the 2022 report, which is publicly available.[2]

Very briefly, some of these suggestions included:

- that the trends could be explained by the UK's *ageing population* – that is, more people have been dying because more people are old. As already explained, this makes no sense because the whole point of calculating *age standardised* mortality rates is, er, to standardise (that is, adjust for) age. Life expectancy calculations also take age into account.
- that the changed rates were influenced by *migration*: in essence, this was about more unhealthy people coming into the country in the relevant time period and impacting on mortality rates. In fact, the opposite is true: we know from lots of evidence that people who have the resources to migrate into the UK tend to have much better health than the resident population – this is known as the 'healthy migrant' effect.[186] If anything, therefore, migration might have masked, rather than exacerbated, the mortality crisis that we have seen since the early 2010s.
- that the stalling of overall improvement in life expectancy just reflects a '*natural limit*': we can't all go on living longer and longer every year. This suggestion makes no sense, for three important reasons: first, life expectancy *did* continue to improve over the same period in other countries like Japan, which has the highest life expectancy of any country in the world; second, as we have already discussed at length, the worst mortality changes have been seen in the poorer parts of the UK, areas where life expectancy is nowhere near any kind of such natural 'ceiling'; third, and related to the last point, in many of those areas life expectancy has actually *decreased*, not just stopped improving.
- that particular '*cohorts*' (groups of people born in particular periods) with certain health issues were driving the trends. This is perhaps the most plausible suggestion of those discussed here, especially as we know that such 'cohort effects' have been shown previously for particular causes of

death like suicide and drug-related causes.[187] On the other hand, as already explained several times in this chapter, changes in death rates have been shown for all age groups over a relatively short time period: thus, people born in many different time periods have been affected. It is therefore unlikely that this is a major cause of the overall changes.

• that the effects were 'artefactual', caused by different *technical/analytical* issues. These included the methods used to calculate age-standardised rates, population denominator issues and other factors. When assessed for the 2022 report, there was simply no viable evidence to support these suggestions.[2]

The 'tragic social consequences' of austerity

In this chapter we have set out the evidence that the principal causes of the changes to life expectancy and mortality rates that we have seen in the UK have been government austerity policies. Of other suggested explanations, previous increases in obesity levels in the UK have been shown to be relevant, but likely account for only a small (possibly very small) proportion of what has happened.

As we discussed earlier, the evidence we have presented is principally statistical in nature. Such 'quantitative' analyses are required in seeking to prove or disprove hypotheses. At the same time, however, a fair criticism of these statistical studies is that, by their nature, they examine numbers, and not the individual human experiences: what it means to live with such levels of poverty and stress that it literally makes you ill. Sometimes we need to understand less about numbers, and more about how people actually feel. This can – and has been – provided by a great many 'qualitative' studies in which the impacts on people's mental health and well-being have been recorded in words, not numbers. A great many studies provide testament to the harrowing effects of austerity policies that have made people desperate, and that have made life difficult to live.[152,154,155,188–191] We included a handful of quotations from just a few such studies earlier in the chapter.

'External' testimonies – from those who observe from the outside – can also be powerful. In 2018 Professor Philip Alston embarked on a tour of parts of Britain in his role as the United Nations' so-called 'special rapporteur' on extreme poverty and human rights. Special rapporteurs are independent experts appointed by the United Nations Human Rights Council to investigate alleged human rights violations. In this case, Professor Alston's remit was to assess 'the extent to which the Government's policies and programmes relating to extreme poverty are consistent with its human rights obligations'. It is telling that the UN saw fit to dispatch such an expert on poverty and human rights to modern-day Britain in the first place, and when the report appeared the following year, it was damning in the extreme.[192] Austerity, Professor Alston wrote, had had 'tragic social consequences': child poverty, food banks and homelessness had all increased massively, life expectancy for the poorest had declined:

> The bottom line is that much of the glue that has held British society together since the Second World War has been deliberately removed and replaced with a harsh and uncaring ethos. … British compassion has been replaced by a punitive, mean-spirited and often callous approach apparently designed to impose a rigid order on the lives of those least capable of coping.[192]

'Punitive', 'mean-spirited', 'callous' actions aimed at those in society who have the least, and who are the least able to manage: Alston's words bring to mind those of the late, Glasgow-based, author and political activist, Cathy McCormack. She described such actions as part of a 'war without bullets': an assault by means of policies (rather than guns) on the lives of the poor.[1]

With specific regard to the changes to social security, Alston said:

> It might seem to some observers that the Department of Work and Pensions has been tasked with designing a digital and sanitized version of the nineteenth century workhouse, made infamous by Charles Dickens, rather than seeking to respond creatively and compassionately to the real needs of those facing widespread economic insecurity in an age of deep and rapid transformation brought about by automation, zero-hour contracts and rapidly growing inequality.[192]

It's worth reflecting that the UN was here describing a department of the UK government – a government that at the same time was stating publicly that it was committed to 'levelling up', that is, to narrowing inequalities in British society.[193] One can only assume they weren't terribly serious about it.

The effects of austerity have been horrific. They have also been utterly unnecessary. To quote Philip Alston one last time, in a country as wealthy as the UK, 'poverty is a political choice'.[192] We don't need to have it; our rulers decided to have it, and to increase it.

Alston's report, alongside all the evidence of the health impacts of austerity that we have presented in this chapter, paint a truly grim picture of the UK in the 21st century. They also beg important additional questions. First, what do we need to do about it? We will address that question explicitly in the final chapter of the book. And second, was it just in the UK that these changes took place? What happened in other countries?

Paul

Paul lives in London, and for many years had worked in Public Relations (PR), earning up to £40,000 per year.[1,2] However, he became ill, and an error with his credit rating meant that he lost his privately rented accommodation in the city. His illness quickly worsened, and he was admitted to hospital.

Luckily for Paul, being admitted to hospital in the UK doesn't generate a large medical bill like it might in the US.[3,4] But without a house to return to, he could not be discharged from hospital for three months while the London borough council tried to find him a place to go to. Paul's diagnosis was ME (commonly known as chronic fatigue syndrome), a condition with few effective treatments, variable severity of symptoms, but that is well known to be triggered by periods of stress.[5]

From his hospital bed, Paul was offered a place in a Brixton hostel until a more permanent solution could be found. However, he was having to use a wheelchair regularly by this point, and needed an accessible house. The council had so little suitable housing that he was told that he would be waiting seven years before accommodation appropriate for his needs became available, and so he instead signed up with a private landlord who specialised in housing for people in receipt of benefits. When Paul did this, the council no longer had an obligation to house him. But the private landlord let him down, and he ended up sleeping in his car.

Paul's car is a Mini. As the name suggests, it's small. Out of housing options, Paul slept in this tiny vehicle for *two years*, with his wheelchair and belongings taking up most of the available space. Understandably, Paul's health was poor for much of this time. Sometimes he was able to walk and use some of the council facilities and services around him, like the local swimming pool to have a shower. At other times he was stuck in his car for days at a time, unable to manoeuvre out his wheelchair.

In the end, the police confiscated his car, and Paul was forced to present himself to the council as homeless. Council officers initially refused to believe he was homeless because his car insurance was registered to his old address. When accommodation was eventually offered, the so-called accessible flat had no lift access despite being three floors up. There were more steps to get into the front door, and the doorway was too narrow for the wheelchair to fit. The house itself was a mess. On initial viewing, the front door had been broken into, it was thick with dirt, and the mattress had bloodstains.

Refusal often offends, and in not accepting this sub-standard accommodation, Paul was once again forced into the spiral of homelessness. For Paul this meant sleeping on the sofas of friends until he had exhausted their goodwill, nights in hostels and night shelters, and even sleeping in a disabled toilet.

Paul's experience is far from unique. As we discussed in Chapter 3, the austerity cuts in local government budgets across the UK generally,[6] but particularly in deprived areas,[7] meant that housing services and the people that needed them, were under attack.[8] Total departmental funding for local authorities was *cut by over half* after 2010.[6] The impact of this is obvious. The number of households in temporary accommodation (usually meaning low quality 'bed and breakfast' provision involving a room without much else in the way of facilities, and often some distance from where people's friends and family live) shot up. In London, it increased by more than 50 per cent between 2010 and 2019. In North West England, the increase was over 300 per cent.[9] And all of that has been directly linked to higher mortality, including from alcohol and drugs as people struggled to cope with a lack of a permanent place to call home.[10]

However, Paul's former life in PR did give him some opportunities. He found that he could get away with sleeping in the terminal building at Heathrow airport without being moved on because he still possessed the large Louis Vuitton bag he had bought with his first big pay cheque many years previously. In the eyes of the security and police staff at the airport, he was a well-paid but tired traveller rather than a homeless man, and they therefore left him to sleep.

By 2018 Paul's ME had become so severe that he could neither talk nor walk. When sent an invitation for an assessment of his disability benefits, he understandably couldn't attend. As a result, all of his benefits were unceremoniously stopped.

Things could have been very different. Given the right support, Paul's condition could have been managed, and he might have been in a position to work again. However, once more, austerity ripped away the safety net that should have been there to help him.

What happened to life expectancy in other countries, and why?

If they don't depend on true evidence, scientists are no better than gossips.

Penelope Fitzgerald, 'The Gate of Angels'[1]

In Chapters 1 and 2 we showed how life expectancy trends have changed in the UK, leading to vast numbers of unnecessary deaths. In Chapter 3 we demonstrated that austerity policies introduced after 2010 in the UK were the most important cause of these changes. In this chapter we broaden our horizons to consider what happened in other countries, asking whether life expectancy trends changed outside the UK and, if so, was austerity responsible?

The chapter is structured as follows. First, the range of countries experiencing changed life expectancy trends and austerity policies is described. Second, the evidence of the impacts of austerity policies at international level is discussed, emphasising its robustness and how the methods used make it clear that austerity has *caused* the changes in life expectancy. Third, patterns for specific groups of countries are highlighted, indicating how the experiences of austerity may have differed across nations, and where other explanations might be important to understand why trends have varied.

Trends in life expectancy and mortality across countries and the role of austerity

Adverse changes in life expectancy and mortality trends since the early 2010s have been seen in many countries. Figure 4.1 shows the trends in mortality rates for a selection of high-income nations. Similar to Figure 2.2, the actual trend is shown with the solid black line, with the dotted line representing the *expected* mortality rates, had the previous trends seen between 1999 and 2010 continued. For almost all of these countries a gap between the actual and the projected mortality trends emerges after 2012. In some countries, such as Australia, the Republic of Ireland and South Korea, mortality continued to improve after 2012, but at a slower rate than in the earlier time period. For other countries, such as Germany, the UK and the US, there was almost no improvement (and in the US, mortality actually worsened). All of this contrasts with Japan, which has not only had the lowest mortality of all the countries, but where rates continued to improve throughout the time period.

In comparison to the high-income countries, the trend in many low- and middle-income countries (LMICs) is much more variable (Figure 4.2). This variability over time means that it is not appropriate to fit a (dotted) projection line in the same way as we have done in Figure 4.1. In some countries, such as Brazil and Ecuador, there have been steady improvements, although these have been quite slow in Brazil. In many other countries, however, including Egypt, Malaysia, Paraguay, Peru and South Africa, there have been periods of both improvement and worsening in mortality, and sometimes these changes have been very rapid. There has been no consistency in the timings of the changes

Figure 4.1: Actual (solid line) and projected (dotted line) mortality rates for selected high-income countries (1999–2001 to 2017–19)*

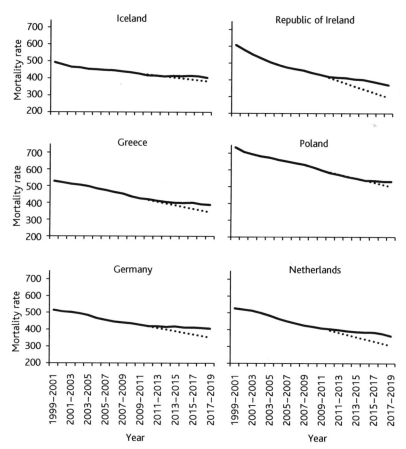

Figure 4.1: Actual (solid line) and projected (dotted line) mortality rates for selected high-income countries (1999–2001 to 2017–19) (continued)

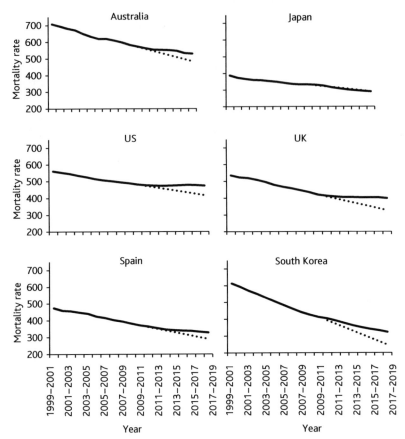

* The mortality data are rolling 3-year average, all-age, age-standardised mortality rates per 100,000 population per year. Countries have been selected to be illustrative of trends in high-income countries rather than comprehensive or representative.

Source: WHO, with the exception of Australia (data obtained from the Australian Bureau of Statistics – standardised to the Australian population), and the Republic of Ireland (which used WHO up to 2011–13 and Eurostat thereafter, interpolating for 2017 and 2018 due to missing data in both sources).

in trends in these countries, suggesting that the widespread 'stalling' or 'stagnation' in life expectancy trends has been limited to richer countries. Further research is needed to better understand whether there are any systematic changes in life expectancy in LMICs, or whether this recent changed trend is restricted to high-income countries. The case studies that follow therefore focus only on high-income countries whose trends are shown in Figure 4.1.

The challenge of assessing and measuring austerity

As we discussed briefly in Chapter 3, there are many different definitions and measures of austerity. This can make it difficult to determine whether or not countries have implemented such policies (and while some countries were open in announcing the adoption of austerity, that was not the case everywhere). It can also hide important differences in the nature of, and context surrounding, austerity: for example, whether austerity was introduced during a period of recession or growth, whether it was based on changes to taxes or spending, which areas of spending were impacted and which social groups were most affected.

Austerity can be defined simply as government policies to cut spending or raise taxes, usually with the intention of increasing economic growth, especially during recession.[2–4] Some ways of identifying and measuring

Figure 4.2: Mortality rates for selected low- and middle-income countries (1999–2001 to 2017–19)*

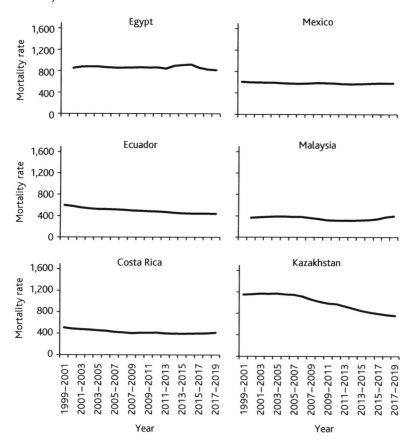

Figure 4.2: Mortality rates for selected low- and middle-income countries (1999–2001 to 2017–19) (continued)

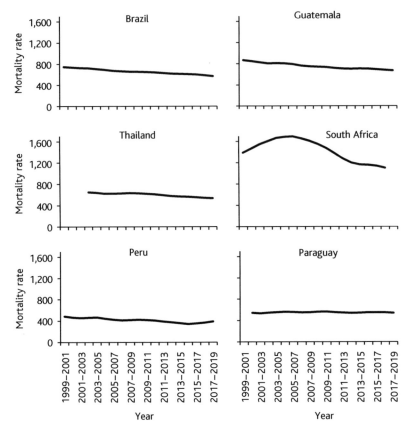

* The mortality data are rolling 3-year average, all-age, age-standardised mortality rates per 100,000 population per year. Countries have been selected to illustrate trends across low- and middle-income countries (LMICs), but are restricted to those with a complete dataset, which biases towards countries with better death-registration systems, and are therefore not representative.

Source: WHO

austerity are more straightforward than others. For example, a simple way is to look at the amount of money spent by governments over time (usually as a percentage of the size of the whole economy) and see if this has reduced. Other measures of austerity look at the balance between taxes and spending to identify whether governments are increasing or reducing the amount of debt they have. The most sophisticated measures look at whether government debt levels are rising or falling after making statistical adjustments for economic growth rates and/or prices.[3,5]

These more complex measures of austerity can be useful for identifying countries where austerity policies have been a deliberate political decision.

For example, an economy in recession will usually see an increase in unemployment, and, with that, government spending on unemployment benefits will increase. At the same time, the amount of money the government takes in taxes will *decrease* because people are earning less and companies are making lower profits. The amount of money taken in by governments during recessions can therefore go down, and the amount of money spent go up, *without any changes to policy*. The changes in taxes and spending which are not a consequence of changes to policy are called 'automatic stabilisers' (these changes are 'automatic' because they don't occur as a result of policy change, and they are 'stabilisers' because they counter the reductions in spending in the economy that result from recession). The more sophisticated measures of austerity generally try to account for these so that the impacts that are due to deliberate changes in policy can be isolated.

However, all measures of austerity – even the more complex ones – are fairly blunt.[3,5] They can identify countries as implementing austerity even when quite different policy approaches are introduced.[6,7] For example, if a government cuts the budget for public services, this will contribute towards lower government spending and might show up as austerity. However, if a government increases taxes (for any group), this will contribute to greater government income, and because this might mean that the government raises more money than it spends, it may also show up as austerity. These measures of austerity therefore don't distinguish between austerity due to changes in taxes or spending, nor do they show which areas of spending are changed, or whether it is the rich or the poor that are impacted more. Another important consideration is that, as mentioned, some of the simpler measures of austerity are calculated as percentages of the size of the economy (for example, gross domestic product [GDP]): thus, two countries which experience the same cuts to public spending might appear very differently on such measures if they have different rates of economic growth. Several of the austerity measures focus on year-to-year changes rather than more stable trends.[8] None of the measures by themselves distinguish between the implementation of austerity during times of economic recession or growth (although some adjust for the rate of economic growth).[5]

The important point here is that most rich countries implemented policies after 2010 which can be described, using these various measures, as austerity.[9] However, this assessment can change, depending on which specific measure of austerity it is based on.[5,9]

Given this complexity, a relatively simple and understandable measure is presented in Figures 4.3–4.6 to identify periods of austerity across countries. It tracks changes in government spending as a percentage of the size of the economy, and therefore focuses attention on times when government spending is cut, or does not keep up with economic growth. However, we also use, and refer to, other, more complicated, measures in our research and assessment of different countries' experiences.

The impacts of austerity across countries

As we have said, the changes to life expectancy and mortality, and widening inequalities in both, have not been confined to the UK.[9-12] Several research studies have demonstrated that countries that implemented austerity policies have experienced slower improvements, or even a worsening, in mortality than countries that have not.[9,13-15] This is important.

Our research of the impact of austerity across countries was the most comprehensive and robust of all the available studies.[9] In that study we estimated the impacts on life expectancy using four different measures of austerity, with separate analyses undertaken of when austerity was implemented during times of economic recession. We included 37 countries in our analyses. We also looked at mortality for different age groups, and for men and women separately. Our research also considered the impacts of austerity on the *variation* in mortality within each country (as a proxy for inequalities in life expectancy). We were able to separate the effects of austerity on life expectancy and mortality from the pre-existing differences between countries, and we checked to make sure that differences in economic growth between countries were not confusing the effects of austerity.[9]

For three of the four measures of austerity we used, the results were clear: the greater the austerity, the worse the life expectancy and mortality trends. The impacts of austerity were seen immediately, with the effects of austerity implemented in any particular year wearing off over time.[9] When the analysis was focused on austerity implemented during periods of economic downturn, the damaging effects on mortality were much larger and were seen across all four austerity measures.[9] This is exactly the situation that affected the UK after 2010, when – as we have discussed – the Conservative-Liberal Democrat governing coalition explicitly introduced austerity policies to reduce government debts by cutting spending on social security benefits and public services.[16] The design of this study allows us to say that the effects are causal because of how we were able to ensure the cause came before the effect, and because we were able to adjust for biases within and between countries, and over time.

In the Appendix we provide a summary table of all the other evidence that demonstrates that austerity has *caused* the change in mortality trends. This includes our international analyses already described, as well as a selection of the studies discussed in Chapter 3, but focusing only on those studies which were numerical and which used sophisticated statistical and methodological techniques to infer a causal relationship between austerity and mortality. A key strength of this evidence base shown in the Appendix is that the studies have arisen from different research groups, using different data, different methods and different countries and time periods. This form of 'triangulation' makes the claim that austerity is an important cause of the changed trends much stronger[17,18] and clearly based on 'true evidence'.[19]

In this book we don't discuss in detail *why* austerity was implemented, and who (if anyone) benefited. This has, however, been discussed by others, most notably the author Mark Blyth.[2] In brief, the primary explicit focus for austerity advocates has been to increase economic growth, and they have argued that reducing government debts and government spending is essential to do that.[20,21] However, the empirical evidence does not support this, and it seems much more likely that austerity is an ideological project designed to lead to lower taxes and spending by governments, which in turn allows for wealthier and more powerful groups to accumulate more.[2,22] Austerity might therefore exacerbate inequalities in power across societies, something that is recognised to exacerbate inequalities in health.[23–25]

In the next section we look at the experiences of particular groups of countries, and assess the extent to which the different forms of austerity implemented in other countries were similar, or different, to that introduced in the UK – and the extent to which that explains different impacts on population health.

Australia, Germany and the Netherlands are discussed as a group because they have all experienced changed life expectancy trends but are not recognised in the public narrative as having implemented austerity. We will show that in fact each of these countries has implemented widespread austerity programmes and that changed trends in life expectancy have resulted.

Following this, the extensive evidence of the change in life expectancy trends in the US is discussed. The US is taken alone because it has undoubtedly the worst trends of rich countries, and it requires particular explanation.

Next, Iceland, Greece, the Republic of Ireland and Spain are discussed as a group, as all had austerity programmes imposed upon them in the aftermath of the 2007/08 financial crisis.

Finally, South Korea and Japan are highlighted as examples of countries that already have very high life expectancy. South Korea has experienced a marked slowdown in the rate of improvement compared to previous trends, whereas Japan has shown consistent improvements across the time period.

Germany, Australia and the Netherlands

Germany, Australia and the Netherlands all experienced stagnating trends in life expectancy after 2012, similar to the UK (Figure 4.1).[9] Using government spending (as percentage of GDP) as the measure of austerity, it can be seen that all four countries have implemented austerity to varying degrees after

Figure 4.3: Exposure to austerity after 2010 in Australia, Germany, Netherlands and the US*

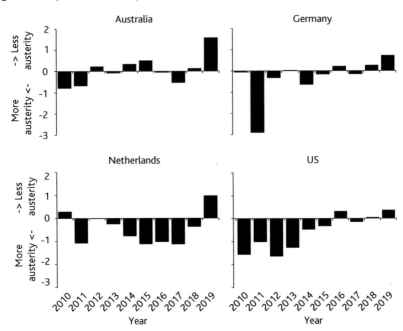

* Measured as the percentage point change in government expenditure as a percentage of GDP from previous year. Note also that the y-axis scales across Figures 4.3–4.5 are different.
Notes: Refer to the notes at the end of this book for a more detailed description.[26]

2010, indicated by the bars below the x-axis in Figure 4.3. The similarities and differences across these countries is discussed in more detail in the following sections.

Germany

Germany is a particularly interesting case study because it has been (wrongly) highlighted as an example of a country that 'disproves' that austerity is a cause of the stalled trends.[27–29] The German government was faced with substantial challenges in the mid-1990s when East and West Germany reunified, and there was a need to invest in a wide range of infrastructure in the East. The government borrowed (and spent) a large amount of money in this period (that is, implemented anti-austerity policies). After 2003, Germany reverted to an austerity approach, albeit in the context of strong economic growth. During the financial crash and immediate recession in 2007–09, the German government again used borrowing to fund public spending, but most measures show that they returned to an austerity approach between 2012 and 2017.[9]

At the start of the COVID-19 pandemic the German government, like almost every government which introduced lockdown measures, had to borrow more money to subsidise affected industries and to support people who could not work.[30] However, this was short lived, and the policy preference for austerity was made clear by the German Economy Minister, Peter Altmaier, in March 2020, when he said, 'Once the [COVID-19] crisis is over – and we hope this will be the case in several months – *we will return to austerity policy*' [emphasis added].[30]

Austerity in Germany was implemented at different governmental levels, and in different ways. Conditions and sanctions for the receipt of social security benefits were increased, disproportionately impacting on immigrant populations. Germany also has, at least until very recently, few routes for immigrants to gain citizenship, creating substantial inequalities in rights and eligibility for people born abroad and ethnic minorities.[31,32]

At local government level, funding was cut across the board and/or charges were increased or introduced.[33,34]

There is no doubt that Germany has experienced changed trends in life expectancy (see Figure 4.1),[9] and that mortality inequalities have increased.[35] However, most interpretations by academics working in Germany have failed to examine the role of economic policy, and have instead focused on descriptive analyses of demographic changes, and speculation about the role of healthcare provision or health behaviours.[10,36–38] Like the UK and US, Germany has eroded its welfare state since the 1990s and privatised key sectors. Protections for workers have been reduced and the real value of benefits has been cut.[39] These policies, widely described as 'neoliberalism', are well known to exacerbate social and health inequalities, and to adversely affect mortality trends.[40,41] It is in this context that further reductions in public spending in Germany have caused stagnation of life expectancy.

Australia

There has been a very similar response from public health academics working in Australia to those in Germany. Stagnating life expectancy trends have been noted, but analysis and interpretation have been limited to the role of changes in particular causes of death and health behaviours, rather than any deeper analysis of the role of social and economic policies.[42,43] As in the other countries in this group, many 'neoliberal reforms' have been introduced in Australia over time,[44] and in the period after 2010 there has been austerity in five of the eight following years although the scale of austerity has been relatively modest on this measure (see Figure 4.3).[9]

Until the 1980s, the Australian economy was characterised by a combination of high levels of regulation and low levels of government ownership. This involved taxes and controls on imports in order to protect Australian industries, compulsory conciliation of disputes between trade unions and business, and national wage bargaining.[44,45] This created the context for low unemployment, high wages and relatively low income inequalities.[44] This policy approach started to change in the early 1980s, and was completely overhauled from 1996 onwards.[44-47]

Between 1996 and 2000 several key economic changes were introduced. First, in common with the UK, the supply of money and the setting of interest rates became the primary means of controlling inflation and unemployment instead of using public spending and tax policy.[44] Second, collective bargaining (that is, when the wages for an entire sector are negotiated between employers and trades unions) was removed and anti-trade union laws were introduced to reduce the power of workers to negotiate for better pay and conditions.[44,45] Third, university education funding was radically changed to a fee-paying model instead of the government-funding approach that had previously existed.[44] Finally, the social security system was changed to introduce conditions on receiving welfare payments (such as obligations to be applying for jobs).[44,48] All of these changes were made in the belief that markets would create faster economic growth, and this growth would spread across the population.[45] Although there was economic growth, there was also an increase in economic inequality and a rise in the number of precarious jobs (that is, jobs without the contract or hours that provide a secure income).[44]

This all meant that by around 2000, the broad direction of Australian economic policy was similar to that in the UK and US, with a small public sector, low regulation and a social security system characterised by low levels of payment and numerous conditions for recipients.

The changes to social security introduced in Australia have marked similarities to those introduced in the UK. The legitimacy of benefit claimants has been questioned by governments and the media, leading to stigmatisation.[49,50] An array of additional hurdles have been introduced which require people to demonstrate need or undertake additional tasks in order to confirm their eligibility.[48,49] This increase in 'conditionality' has contributed to widening inequalities, particularly impacting on First Nation peoples.[49] One example of this approach is termed 'Compulsory Income Management', which restricts access to welfare payments for those unable to demonstrate 'responsible behaviours',[49] similar to the UK's benefit sanction approach. Shame, discrimination, racism, social isolation and disempowerment have all been reported as a result.[49]

The changes to social security and economic policy are therefore closely associated with the changed trends in average life expectancy shown in Figure 4.1. It has also exacerbated existing ethnic health inequalities. As in most other high-income countries, life expectancy in Australia had been increasing on average in the decades before the 2010s. However, inequalities in health are large between socioeconomic groups,[51] and between the non-Indigenous population and Aboriginal and Torres Strait Islander peoples.[52]

The latter inequalities are a direct product of colonisation and discriminatory government policies over a prolonged period, resulting in life expectancy being 8.6 years and 7.8 years lower for Aboriginal and Torres Strait Islander males and females, respectively, by 2015–17.[52]

The Netherlands

Following a now familiar pattern, the changed mortality and life expectancy trends in the Netherlands have been subject to only the most superficial analyses. It is clear that life expectancy improvements have stalled (see Figure 4.1), and that inequalities are widening.[10,11,53,54] However, research has focused on specific causes of death such as influenza, and on the role of health behaviours,[54,55] with no investigation of the impact of economic policies despite the clear implementation of austerity (see Figure 4.3).[33,56–61] Although inequalities in mortality by ethnicity have long been recognised in the Netherlands,[62,63] there are few available data to know if the recent widening in socioeconomic inequalities has impacted on particular ethnic groups disproportionately.

In common with Australia, Germany and the UK, the Netherlands has transitioned its economic and social policies since the 1990s towards less generous social security, increased privatisation and reduced public sector service provision.[64] Labour laws were changed to reduce the power of trade unions and to restrict access to unemployment benefits, increasing the number of jobs which are precarious.[58] Despite legal protections against discrimination, racism is still widely experienced and anti–immigration politicians have gained substantial support in recent years.[65–68]

Unlike some other countries in the eurozone, the Netherlands actually had relatively low levels of government debt in 2010 (the reduction of government debt is often used as a rationale for austerity policies, as some economists argue that debt impedes economic growth).[60] Nevertheless, the pursuit of austerity was at least as aggressive here as it was in other countries in Europe that had much higher levels of debt,[60,61] with austerity implemented every year from 2011 and 2018 (see Figure 4.3). These austerity policies are estimated to have reduced the size of the economy by around an additional 3 per cent between 2011 and 2013, and (somewhat ironically) to have substantially increased government debt as a result.[60]

Between 2011 and 2018 austerity was implemented across a range of spending areas, with increases in the age of retirement, cuts to long-term social care and the replacement of student scholarships with student loans.[58] After adjusting for inflation, local government (municipality) spending in the Netherlands decreased by 12 per cent between 2010 and 2015, similar in scale to some parts of the UK (as we discussed in Chapter 3).[57] Implementing the cuts, the Dutch government sought to frame austerity as an opportunity for civic organisations (for example, the voluntary sector) to provide more of the services and infrastructure in communities. This was termed the 'Participation Society', akin to the UK government's narrative of the 'Big Society' (which suggested that local volunteers could provide support in lieu of public services).[57] At local level, austerity was implemented through a combination of service cuts and price increases, but also through changes to how services were delivered.[33] One example of this is social care for older adults, where long-term social care accommodation was cut by 40 per cent over two years, with the expectation that this care would instead be provided in the community by family members and existing social networks.[59] This led to gaps in social care for lower-income groups who were unable to afford to pay for social care services.[59]

The case of the US

The case of the US is important to understand because, for what is the richest nation on earth, life expectancy trends have been, frankly, appalling. Figure 4.1 shows that life expectancy in the US has not just stagnated but actually *declined* in the years immediately after 2013.[10,11] What makes this even more shocking is that life expectancy in the US was already comparatively very low. Up until the late 1970s, life expectancy in the US was similar to other wealthy countries and was improving at a similar rate.[69] However, after 1980 the rate of improvement slowed, as compared to other countries, such that by 2010 the US had one of the lowest life expectancies of all high-income countries.[69-71] So, what happened in the 1980s to change these trends?

The shift to neoliberalism in the 1980s

In 1981 Ronald Reagan was elected president and introduced a new economic model over the course of the 1980s. This new model mirrored changes introduced in the UK by Margaret Thatcher, and the economic approach promoted across the world by international financial agencies such as the International Monetary Fund.[41,72-74] This 'neoliberal' economic model has several features, all of which promote the use of markets in the economy. First, taxes for the rich and for businesses were reduced. Second, there was greater tolerance of unemployment, not least because this was intended to reduce demands from workers for higher wages. Third, social security benefits were reduced in value and greater conditions were put in place for their receipt. Fourth, various aspects of the economy were privatised. Finally, public spending on many services was squeezed (with the notable exception of military expenditure, which was increased substantially).[75-78] Somewhat ironically, the net result of these policies was the opposite of austerity, as the large tax cuts and rise in unemployment increased government deficits, reduced the amount of money raised by the US government and increased the amount of money spent.[79] However, the policies also led to a rapid increase in income and wealth inequalities, an erosion of public services and social security and an increasingly divided country.[80,81]

The slower rate of life expectancy improvement between 1980 and 2010 in the US has been directly linked to this changed economic model.[41,41,82,83] Much of the change in life expectancy at this time was due to increased inequalities in mortality.[84] This increasing mortality inequality was mirrored by widening geographical gaps across the country, with mortality becoming much higher in rural areas, particularly in the South–Central and Mid–West counties, compared to other areas.[85]

From bad to worse: life expectancy trends after 2010

After around 2010, this already bad situation became markedly worse, with – as stated – life expectancy decreasing after 2013 (see Figure 4.1).[10,69,86–88] This change in life expectancy was more extreme than in other countries, but occurred around the same time.[9,11]

In contrast to most other countries (with the notable exception of the UK), the falling life expectancy trends in the US have been the subject of substantial research activity and debate. A comprehensive review of the causes of the recent decline in life expectancy highlighted a series of contributing factors.[89,90]

First, the role of 'neoliberal' policies, which have eroded the social security system, reduced access to healthcare services, reduced the rights of workers, reduced spending on public services and infrastructure, and which have created one of the most unequal of all rich countries, was emphasised.[91–93] This is important in understanding why the US population has been more vulnerable to subsequent policy changes,[94] but also provides context to the range of more specific political choices that have had such devastating health consequences.

Second, many policies which are important for population health are decided at state level in the US, rather than federal level. This includes some aspects of worker rights, minimum pay legislation, the regulation of harmful substances such as tobacco and alcohol, some aspects of migration policy, civil rights, healthcare provision (see later) and gun control.[95,96] In recent years policy changes across these areas have generally damaged health, through reductions in the rights of workers, loosening of the regulation of harmful substances, erosion of civil rights, restrictions in the funding of and access to public healthcare, and loosening of gun control.[90] The trends have not been uniform across states, but it has been estimated that, in combination, they have reduced life expectancy for the US overall by 2.8 years for women and 2.1 years for men.[96]

The problems with the US healthcare system are particularly noteworthy. It is one of the most expensive healthcare systems in the world, yet millions of people do not have access to the care they need.[97-99] The private insurance model is costly, with huge administrative costs which waste resources[100] ('transaction costs' – the processes of estimating prices, billing and managing insurance risk – are estimated to account for *one quarter* of all US healthcare spending[101]). There are few mechanisms in place to stop money being spent on treatments and medications that don't work (unlike in the UK), and the systems in place to prevent ill-health and promote positive health (for example, smoking–cessation programmes) are very weak by international standards.[102-104] The US healthcare system is arguably an example of what has been called 'state capture':[105] this is where an industry is able to make undue and large profits from the government because of a lack of independent regulation and control – in the case of the US, this is made possible by powerful lobby groups and their funding of political parties.[104,106-108] Although there have been some attempts to broaden access to healthcare for the public, implementation has been limited,[109] not least because of the power of individual states to block this.[96] These ongoing problems with the quality of and access to US healthcare are an important contributor to the falling life expectancy.[90] Indeed, it is estimated that *a quarter* of the US's higher mortality as compared to other countries between the ages of 18 and 64 years (45,000 deaths per year) was due to an absence of universal healthcare.[110]

Third, after 2010, inequalities in income and wealth continued to grow in the US,[111] despite the country already being one of the most unequal of all rich countries.[80] The most important contributor to this was a rapid rise in the income and wealth of people who were already rich – the top 1 per cent. Indeed, Oxfam has calculated that in 2022 the US had 735 billionaires (that is, people with *wealth at least 1,000 times greater than a millionaire*).[112] Given the known negative impacts of economic inequalities on the health of populations (as they widen health inequalities and bring down average life expectancy),[40] this has been another important contributor to the decline in US life expectancy after 2010.[90] One reason for the wide economic inequalities in the US is the 'stinginess' of welfare benefits. These are much lower than in most other rich countries, and therefore mean that more people cannot afford the basic necessities for staying healthy. It has been calculated that US life expectancy would be 3.8 years longer if the generosity of the welfare state matched the average for other wealthy countries.[113]

Economic inequalities in the US exist not just between different social classes, but between Black, Hispanic, Asian, Indigenous and White populations. Mortality rates are substantially higher among Black and Indigenous populations. This is caused by systemic and structural racism, where laws, institutions and the dominant culture discriminate against particular groups and impact on all of the 'social determinants of health' discussed in Chapter 3.[82,114–116] It has historical roots in colonialism and slavery, but has continued to be evident in some laws and institutional practices ever since (exemplified by the murder of George Floyd by US law-enforcement officers in 2020).[116–118] The more recent rise in racism facilitated by the Trump presidency has simply exacerbated these damaging effects on health.[119,120]

Fourth, although trends have worsened for almost all causes of death, drug-related deaths in particular have increased very quickly, especially among the working-age population.[87,88,121] The evidence shows that this increase is related to changes in both the supply of illicit drugs and the demand for them.[121] The over-prescribing of oxycontin and fentanyl (two commonly misused opioids) in the US healthcare system, not least because of the actions of the pharmaceutical industry[107] and a lack of adequate regulation, have been important in making illicit drugs more widely available.[121] On the other side, the demand for illicit drugs has also increased, not least because of all of the social and economic disruption, and associated 'despair',[87] described earlier. In addition, increases in physical pain, mental ill-health and the experience of adversity (such as parental separation, imprisonment and abuse) have all increased the demand for illicit drugs.[121]

Mortality from suicide has also increased markedly in the US.[87] Many of the causes of suicide are similar to the causes of drug-related deaths. However, suicide (and homicide) are also influenced by the availability of firearms, regulation of which is lower in the US as compared to other countries.[90]

Drug-related deaths and suicide have had substantial publicity as important causes of declining life expectancy,[87] but the diseases that kill most people are the same as they are in other rich countries.[122] Cardiovascular disease (which, as we described in the last chapter, includes heart attacks, strokes and many of the consequences of diabetes) and cancers are responsible for most of the declining life expectancy. These specific causes of death are the end point of the economic and social divisions described earlier, and operate through the same stress-related 'causal pathways' described in detail in Chapter 3. However, they are also related to the large rise in the proportion of the US population who are obese, which is in turn related to changes in the food system and physical environment (which is discussed in more detail in Chapter 6).[90] It is estimated that 55 per cent of the difference in life expectancy between the US and other countries can be explained by higher levels of obesity.[123]

Austerity in the US

What is missing from public health experts' current range of explanations for the changes to life expectancy trends after 2010 in the US is the impact of austerity policies.[10,124] To a large degree this is because 'austerity' is neither a common political framing within the US, nor a new policy direction.[82,116] In many ways, the US population has been subject to the policies of austerity for a very long time, and whenever public spending has increased, it has been spent on the military or on attempts to mitigate the problems created by the country's broken and vastly unequal economic system (for example, on prisons and policing).

More recently, the extent of austerity in the US has been reported to be larger than in the UK, with substantial reductions in the fiscal deficit having taken place between 2010 and 2013 (see Figure 4.3).[125] This was due to restrictions imposed by the Republican-controlled Congress, which passed the Budget Control Act to control spending.[126] It is also important to note that budget bills have been used to reduce federal funding for social security and the Internal Revenue Service (which prevents tax evasion), while protecting or increasing military expenditure.[127]

The impacts of austerity are likely to depend not only on the scale of the economic changes implemented within any particular country, but on the degree to which the population is vulnerable to such changes. For example, if employment within a particular country is dominated by a particular sector (such as making cars), it might flourish while the demand for those cars continues and the sector continues to provide well-paid work. However, if circumstances change to mean that the jobs are moved elsewhere or demand for those cars disappears, the *vulnerability* of the population is revealed, and can have disastrous consequences.[94] It is well known that the US has a series of vulnerabilities that have been revealed since 2010. This includes the very basic welfare protections for its citizens, which has left millions of people with no access to healthcare and other essentials,[128–130] ongoing structural racism and discrimination, which is most obviously seen through police brutality,[115,116] stark inequalities, political polarisation, challenges to democracy and the opioid crisis.

The US therefore has suffered the 'perfect storm' of pre-existing vulnerability as a consequence of four decades of neoliberalism, compounded by structural racism, rising inequalities and austerity.[90,116] It is no wonder that US life expectancy has fallen.

Iceland, Greece, Spain and the Republic of Ireland

Iceland, Greece, Spain and the Republic of Ireland are a group of countries which, following the financial crash in 2007/08, had austerity imposed upon them, to varying degrees, by international institutions such as the European Central Bank and International Monetary Fund.[131,132] As such, there was substantial early concern from researchers that life expectancy trends in these countries would falter.[133,134] This section discusses the experience of austerity (Figure 4.4) and life expectancy trends (see Figure 4.1) in each of these countries in turn.

Figure 4.4: Exposure to austerity after 2010 in Iceland, Greece, the Republic of Ireland and Spain*

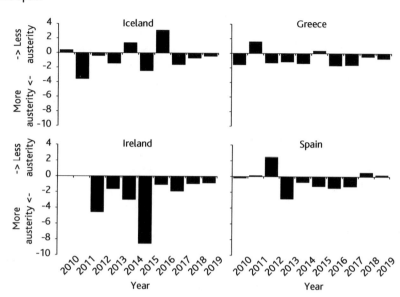

* Measured as the percentage point change in government expenditure as a percentage of GDP from the previous year. Note also that the y-axes across Figures 4.3–4.5 are different. Data for Ireland in 2010 and 2011 were not available.

Iceland

As recently as the mid–20th century, Iceland was one of the poorest countries in Europe. However, the privatisation and deregulation of the banking and finance sector during the 1980s led to rapid economic growth.[135] The extent of the reorientation of the Icelandic economy towards financial speculation is hard to overestimate. In early 2007, Iceland's three largest banks had assets worth *eight times the total annual income of Iceland*.[135] However, this economic model was built on sand, with most of this wealth ultimately being found to be near worthless, bought with borrowed money rather than real assets.[135–137] These private banks made Iceland more vulnerable than many other countries to the financial crisis in 2007/08,[138] and several banks collapsed because a high proportion of loans they had made were defaulted upon.[135,136]

Although the financial sector followed a neoliberal model, taxation was used to redirect some of this income into both a generous social security system and high–quality public services.[135] Income inequality had risen during the 1990s and 2000s, but it remained at much lower levels than in most other rich countries because of the social policy measures that had been pursued.[139]

Iceland received a financial bailout from the International Monetary Fund (IMF) in 2009, one of the conditions for which was the implementation of austerity measures (evidenced by the bars below the x-axis in Figure 4.4).[138] The financial crisis and subsequent austerity led to a substantial decline in the size of the economy, with GDP dropping by 7 per cent.[138] However, the nature of the austerity implemented in Iceland was quite different to that implemented in the UK.[140] This different approach was arguably in direct response to vocal mass protests which demanded that those responsible for the financial crisis should pay, not the wider public.[141-143]

The banks were nationalised and split into domestic and foreign arms, and the bankers responsible were prosecuted for financial crimes.[138] Many of the unpayable debts of Icelandic citizens were erased, including mortgage loans.[138] The currency was allowed to decline substantially in value to make exports more competitive, and 'capital controls' – to prevent large-scale movements of money in and out of the country – were introduced.[138]

Taxes were increased, but only for richer people, and social security benefits were protected.[138] However, there were cuts to health services[140] and education, and public sector pay was reduced.[138] The cuts led to shortfalls in service provision, with people unable to obtain the health and social care they needed.[144] Deprivation and poverty trends for children living in Iceland were relatively stable between 2004 and 2014, with some short-lived declines.[140,145] However, because average incomes fell, the 'poverty line' also decreased (as it is calculated as a percentage of average incomes), and so, while people's living standards declined, that decline was felt across society rather than just in the poorest groups.[146]

The Icelandic austerity experience is therefore somewhat mixed. In some ways the burden of austerity was placed on richer groups, with higher taxes and (although not an economic intervention) the prosecution of bankers. Key social security measures were protected and unpayable mortgage debts were erased. However, real incomes for the poorest groups declined, and health and education services were cut.

Mortality trends in Iceland have not been good, with a notable change in the overall trend (see Figure 4.1). The stalling in Iceland has been less than in many other countries, but the population is small and there are marked fluctuations over time, and so interpretation needs to cautious. Most measures of child health are continuing to improve.[147] The cuts to health and education services, and the decline in real incomes for the poorest groups, are both likely to be important in explaining the changes. However, it also seems likely that some of the policy responses will have protected the population against what might have been even worse consequences.

Greece

Arguably, Greece was the country upon which the most severe austerity measures were imposed by international financial organisations after the financial crisis in 2007/08.[131,148] However, this is not entirely clear from the data on changes to government expenditure as a percentage of GDP (austerity again being represented by the bars below the x-axis in Figure 4.4), not least because the Greek economy contracted so substantially and consistently in the years after 2010 that expenditure would have had to have fallen very fast to keep up with the decreases in GDP.[149] At the start of the crisis, Greece spent among the lowest of all European countries on social expenditure (<15 per cent of GDP), and thus had one of the most limited economic safety nets for its population.[150]

The first financial bailout received by Greece in 2010 came with a requirement to raise €80 billion by mid-2013 through a combination of spending cuts and tax increases. The second bailout required €130 billion of budget reductions to be introduced by 2015, and the third bailout €86 billion by 2018.[151] One condition of the financial bailouts of Greece was rapid and widespread weakening of both worker protections and collective bargaining for higher wages.[152] The minimum wage requirements for workers were also reduced,[152] and wage levels duly declined.[153] Unemployment also increased markedly.[153]

Health services in Greece were also targeted for cuts, with their budget up to 2014 almost halved.[149] There was a rapid increase in the number of people without healthcare insurance, largely because of the rise in unemployment.[148] The range of health services that required patients to pay (for example, to visit a general practitioner [family doctor] or to obtain prescribed medicine), and the price of existing medical payments, all increased.[148] This meant that the relative gap in the amount of healthcare that people needed, but didn't receive, increased ten-fold between the richest and poorest groups.[154] Cuts in the services provided to drug users, including the provision of clean needles, may have caused an HIV (human immunodeficiency virus) outbreak,[148,155] although the numbers are disputed.[156] Suicides also increased.[157,158]

Local government expenditure in Greece was slashed between 2008 and 2015, dropping by 25 or 30 per cent, depending on the data used.[159] The scale of local government cuts was the second-greatest in Europe, dwarfed only by that implemented in Ireland (and possibly Hungary) over this time.[159] A wide range of public assets (for example, ports) were also privatised as part of the austerity package, creating a drain of resources from the Greek government to (usually) foreign owners.[131]

It is no surprise, therefore, given the widespread cuts to services, the rise in unemployment and the increases in costs to people who were already experiencing declining incomes, that overall life expectancy trends stagnated in Greece and, in some years, declined (see Figure 4.1).

Republic of Ireland

The Republic of Ireland was a relatively poor country on the periphery of Europe for much of the 20th century. From the late 1990s it experienced rapid economic growth, catching up with the rest of Europe, and earning it the moniker of the 'Celtic Tiger'.[160] Much of this growth was based on a 'neoliberal' restructuring of the economy, including the use of low corporation tax rates and access to European Union (EU) markets to attract large international companies to base themselves in the country (particularly banks).[161]

In Ireland, many public services, including many aspects of healthcare, are paid for through private insurance schemes and direct payments. The Irish approach is therefore characterised by welfare payments to those in need, but limited provision of public services by government.[161] Direct taxes on incomes and profits were reduced during the 1990s, with much of the government's income coming from taxes on 'capital gains' (that is, money made simply from owning assets such as land when prices are rising), and taxes on land and housing sales. This meant that government income dropped dramatically at the time of the financial crisis as these dried up.[161]

Rapid economic growth and immigration from across the EU led to increases in house prices and substantial financial speculation in the 2000s.[161] This left the Republic with a set of banks with bad debts when the financial crisis hit in 2007/08. House prices and demand for construction collapsed, leading to a deep recession.[161] As in the cases of other EU governments experiencing financial problems, international financial institutions mandated austerity measures in response.[131,161,162]

The scale of austerity introduced between 2008 and 2015 was large, totalling €20.5 billion of spending cuts and €11.5 billion of tax increases, equating to approximately 20 per cent of Irish GDP.[162] The scale of austerity in Figure 4.4 looks greater in Ireland than in Iceland, Greece or Spain; however, this is because it is skewed by economic growth having been much faster here than in those other countries.

In addition to the cuts in spending and increases in taxation, several conditions were placed on the Irish government in order for them to receive financial support from international financial organisations. These included legislative changes to reduce both minimum wages and the power of trade unions to negotiate wages, as well as increased conditions on welfare payments, including sanctions on unemployment benefits.[150,162–164] The immediate spending cuts involved: pay cuts of 5–20 per cent for public sector workers; a pension tax averaging 7 per cent; and reductions in the size of the public sector workforce achieved through early retirements, career breaks and a policy of not filling vacancies.[164] However, the full range of conditions for the financial bailout was not fully implemented.[162] The 'Croke Park Agreement' between trade unions and governments meant that public services would be restructured to cut costs, but that there would be no further pay cuts or compulsory redundancies after the initial cuts already listed.[164]

The public sector workforce was cut by 8 per cent between 2008 and 2015, with services 'reformed' through outsourcing, digitalisation, privatisation and sharing of functions across agencies.[159,164] Local government was hit hardest, with a 23 per cent cut in workers, and a widespread merger of local democratic institutions into larger bodies (for example, town councils were merged into municipalities and city councils, and there was a reduction in numbers of elected councillors).[164] Central and local government capital spending (that is, on replacing or repairing infrastructure) was cut by more than half.[159,165]

Spending cuts impacted on voluntary and community organisations with a particular focus on community development, social inclusion and social housing.[166–168] There is also evidence that more people who needed healthcare were unable to access it.[169] Within higher education a series of changes were introduced, including privatisation and casualisation of employment contracts (that is, moving people onto temporary or 'zero-hours' contracts).[170] Ironically, however, more detailed accounts of where and how austerity was implemented are not available because the researchers and independent organisations who would have undertaken this work had their funding and positions cut.[171]

Unemployment trebled between 2007 and 2012, before subsequently falling.[172,173] However, much of that subsequent fall is accounted for by the emigration of 610,000 people between 2008 and 2015.[173] These were predominantly highly educated young people seeking graduate-level jobs that were no longer available at home.[173]

Economic inequalities and poverty were kept at pre-financial-crisis levels through the use of taxes and social security payments (for example, through short-term increases in unemployment benefits[165]) to redistribute incomes.[174,175] The pre-crisis generosity of the social security system in the Republic of Ireland, and its broad maintenance despite other austerity policies, is in stark contrast to some other countries such as Greece and Spain. In 2009, social expenditure was around 60 per cent of GDP in the Republic of Ireland, compared to around 38 per cent in Greece, and around 28 per cent in Spain.[165] Social security payments were largely protected (and unemployment benefits increased), and poverty and income inequality levels remained steady.

It has been argued that, in contrast to the form of austerity implemented in Iceland, the Irish approach to austerity has protected the wealth of the rich and maintained the country's tax-haven status, while also reducing provision for some marginalised groups, reducing public sector pay and increasing unemployment.[175,176] However, strong economic growth after 2013 allowed for some restoration of pay and a small increase in the public sector workforce,[162,164] again in contrast to Spain and (especially) Greece.[152,165] This seems to have been possible in Ireland because of ongoing demand for Irish exports (and foreign direct investment[177]), facilitated by its open economy.[165] The distinctive nature of austerity in Ireland, including its particular ability to force through large public sector pay cuts[152] and the incredible dominance of exports in the economy (at over 100 per cent of GDP, compared to around 30–40 per cent for Greece and Spain),[152] led one academic to comment that: 'Ireland is not a poster child for austerity but rather a beautiful freak.'[165]

Although mortality has continued to improve in the Republic of Ireland since 2010, it has improved much more slowly than previously (see Figure 4.1), especially for women.[178] Suicides increased for men by 57 per cent in the 2008–12 period, but were unchanged for women.[179] Overall, the protection of the social security system in Ireland, and the export-orientated growth that helped to mitigate public spending cuts after 2013, might have contributed to the continued improvements in mortality. However, the austerity that was implemented still seems to have had a markedly damaging impact, leaving mortality much higher than it would have been had the pre-2010 trends continued (see Figure 4.1).

Spain

Spain shares many of the same characteristics of Greece and Ireland in its experience of rapid growth in construction and broader economic growth in the years leading up to the 2007/08 financial crisis.[152] This left it very vulnerable as credit became more expensive, and the Spanish government quickly found itself with a large budget deficit and unsustainable debts. As is the case in Iceland and Greece, the cuts in government expenditure as a percentage of GDP do not look large (again, represented by the bars below the x-axis in Figure 4.1), but this is because GDP decreased so much, meaning that government spending would have had to have dropped very quickly to keep up with declining GDP.

The austerity package implemented in Spain from around 2009 was very similar to that in Greece.[152] Public sector pay and pensions were cut.[152] Social security benefits were reduced for those who were unemployed, and the retirement age was increased.[152] Spending on education was cut, as was the size of the civil service.[152] A series of policies reduced workers' rights, including the removal of sectoral pay bargaining.[152] Unemployment increased rapidly from under 10 per cent in 2007 to around 25 per cent in 2013.[152] Local government spending was cut between 2008 and 2015, but to a smaller degree than in Ireland or Greece.[159]

The impact of austerity on mortality in Spain was to decrease the rate of improvement. The trends are therefore better than in the US or UK, and similar to that seen in Greece (see Figure 4.1). The slightly different mortality trends and experiences of austerity across these countries highlight the need for research to better understand and compare the *nature* of the austerity implemented across countries.

Japan and South Korea

Japan and South Korea are examples of countries which already had very high levels of life expectancy, but which also experienced continuing improvements after 2012. Korea did have a marked slowdown in the rate of improvement after 2011, leaving mortality rates worse than they would have been, had the previous trends continued (see Figure 4.1); however, rates still declined throughout the period.

Japan did not introduce an austerity programme in the period from 2010, with changes of less than one percentage point in the measure we show in Figure 4.5 in almost every year. Korea did cut government expenditure as a percentage of GDP by almost 2 per cent in 2010, and retained this for around eight years, before reversing that cut. Relative to many of the other countries discussed, however, the scale of austerity in Korea was modest.

Japan had experienced a prolonged period of low or zero economic growth with deflation of its currency during the 1990s and 2000s.[180] The country has notably low levels of income inequality, due to low wage inequality as compared to other rich countries, although it doesn't have a generous social security system.[181,182] Given this underlying low level of inequality, and the absence of austerity measures, it is no surprise that mortality continued to improve at the same rate as before 2010.

The experience of Japan demonstrates that stagnating life expectancy trends are not inevitable in richer countries, and that alternative economic policies have different impacts on mortality. This is particularly important because of the suggestions discussed in Chapter 3 that life expectancy had

Figure 4.5: Exposure to austerity after 2010 in Japan and Korea*

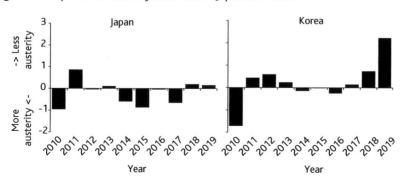

* Measured as the percentage point change in government expenditure as a percentage of GDP from the previous year. Note also that the y-axes across Figures 4.3–4.5 are different.

reached its 'natural limit' in some countries (despite the stalled or declining trends being generally worse in the more socioeconomically disadvantaged groups across countries which already had lower life expectancies).

Korea, on the other hand, has high levels of income and wealth inequality, and high levels of poverty.[183] Like Japan, it does not have a generous social security system, relying instead on private insurance schemes and social care provision by families.[129,182] Even a (relatively) small degree of austerity in Korea has been sufficient to markedly slow the rate of mortality improvement, probably because of this underlying vulnerability related to its high inequality levels.

Conclusion

This chapter has discussed the austerity and life expectancy trends in selected wealthy countries around the world, allowing us to draw out several important lessons. First, the stagnating trends in life expectancy have been seen in many high-income countries, but not all. LMICs have experienced much more variable trends, with periods of rapid improvement and rapid worsening, and no clear patterning emerging.

Second, among high-income countries, austerity policies were not restricted to the UK (and note that the chart for the UK is shown for comparison in Figure 4.6 below). Rather, these were widely implemented, including in countries such as Germany which have been held up as examples of why austerity is not responsible for the changes to mortality rates in the UK.

Third, there is good evidence at international level that those countries which implemented greater austerity (defined in different ways), had worse life expectancy and mortality trends than those that did not, and that these trends were even worse when austerity was implemented at times of economic downturn.

Figure 4.6: Exposure to austerity after 2010 in the UK

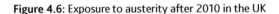

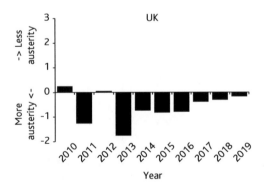

Fourth, the underlying strength of the welfare state, including the generosity of the social security system and the availability and quality of public services, is likely to be important in understanding why the impacts of austerity have been worse in some countries than others. It is clear that some nations, most notably the US, have populations which are particularly vulnerable to economic shocks and austerity policies because of the threadbare nature of the welfare state, wide inequalities and widespread structural racism.

Fifth, there has been considerable variety in the nature of austerity policies implemented across countries, including differences in the balance between cuts to public services, increases in taxes, increases in service charges and privatisations. Another crucial consideration is which social groups have been most impacted by austerity, including whether increased burdens have been placed on richer or poorer groups.[2,6,29,133,184,185] The different type of austerity implemented, and the extent to which the most vulnerable groups were protected, are likely to have mattered for mortality trends.

The next chapter refocuses on the UK, discussing how people responsible for the health of populations, including governments and public health agencies, responded to the data on the changed life expectancy trends and the evidence of the causal role of austerity policies.

Moira

When it began in 2010, the Conservative-Liberal Democrat coalition's austerity programme was accompanied by a highly successful[1-5] policy of vilification and demonisation of people in receipt of social security benefits.[6-10] Promoted by the government to help justify cuts of tens of billions of pounds from social security budgets,[11] and amplified enthusiastically by large sections of the media, it effectively resulted in a considerable proportion of the UK population being portrayed as a collective work-shy drain on national resources. Rather than highlighting the hardship of being less well off or dealing with disability in the face of cuts to income, tabloid headlines instead screamed of cheats and fraudsters, scroungers and skivers.[6,9,10]

Research has effectively demonstrated the baseless claims that were incorporated into this narrative.[12] And it's hard to think of someone to whom the term 'skiver' could be more inappropriately applied than Moira Drury.

Moira was born in Glasgow in the 1950s. Her father owned a window-cleaning business in the city. When Moira was just five years old, the family – Moira, her parents and four siblings – upped sticks and relocated to the English Midlands. Settled in England, Moira excelled at school: head girl, and proud recipient of a Duke of Edinburgh Gold Award. On leaving school, she trained and qualified as a nurse. She was immensely proud of the profession, and of her role in it.

By the 1980s she was married with three young children, and working in a West Midlands hospital. Her husband was abusive, however, frequently beating her, and taking her money. In 1983 Moira was the victim of an unimaginably horrific assault: her husband attempted to kill her, attacking her from behind with a sledgehammer while their three daughters slept upstairs. Moira was hospitalised with severe head injuries. Her husband was sent to jail.[13,14]

Such injuries are traumatic and long lasting. Discharged from hospital, Moira was left with epilepsy, weakness on the left side of her head and depression: understandably, it was not just her physical health that had been affected. Yet, despite all this, she refused to sign on for the sickness benefits to which she was fully entitled. Instead she returned to work night shifts in the hospital to support her young family – now as a single parent.

It was a real struggle for her, but she wanted to continue working in her chosen caring profession.

While Moira did later take time out to care for her three girls (and to further her own recovery), she then returned to work, and was employed for many years as a hospital receptionist. However, in 2007 things caught up with her. By then in her early 50s, her health was deteriorating: alongside the epilepsy, she had experienced two transient ischaemic attacks ('mini strokes') was struggling to walk, suffering from severe depression and in cognitive decline. Moira was forced to give up work.[13,14]

In early 2015, as the UK government ramped up its austerity programme and more and more cuts to social security came into force,[15,16] Moira's benefits were stopped. She had failed to attend an interview to determine whether she was well enough to work – on the fairly reasonable grounds that she was extremely unwell. A letter from the Department for Work and Pensions (DWP) effectively stated that diarrhoea, diabetes and epilepsy were not good enough reasons to miss her appointment.[13,17]

Moira was then sucked into a bureaucratic whirlpool of confusion and miscommunication. A system that had quickly and efficiently cut off her income proved less efficient when it came processing a reapplication for benefit and informing Moira of the possibility of an appeal. The results of this were: no money to live on, a huge amount of health-damaging stress and further, deep, depression. The final straw came after six months of relentless, stress-inducing misery: a court summons arrived for non-payment of her council tax. With the withdrawal of her disability benefit by the DWP, the local council had automatically stopped her council tax benefit as well. The bill for almost £2,000 arrived the same day that she was diagnosed with a further health problem – lung cancer.

Moira was now terminally ill. But even that was not enough to satisfy the DWP. One of her daughters, Nichole, was told in a 'cruel and heartless' phone call that they would not believe Moira was terminally ill unless they were told by a doctor that she only had a few weeks left to live. They had requested evidence from the general practitioner (GP), they said. The GP told Nichole they had received no such request.

In August 2015, one month after her cancer diagnosis, Moira died. She was 61 years old.

Despite the best attempts of the system to prevent Moira being provided with the financial support to which she was legally entitled, an appeal against the DWP was eventually won, and the backdated payments were made. By then, however, Moira had already passed away. Nichole donated the money to a disability charity. A few months later, another letter arrived from the DWP, inviting Moira to another interview to assess her ability to work.

(Nichole complained to her local Member of Parliament about everything that had happened. The complaint was passed on to the then Minister of State for Employment in the DWP, Priti Patel. She said that she was satisfied with the way that Moira's case had been handled.)

Nichole describes her Mum as 'an amazing lady – incredibly determined, resilient, strong and warm-hearted'. And in some ways, Moira's story is an inspiring one: that same resilience, combined with her pride, meant that she did not ask for any help from the state until she so desperately needed it. When asked, however, the state's response was nothing less than appalling and heartless. In Nichole's words, it is a 'crude and cruel' system, a system which targets 'the most vulnerable, the "low hanging fruit" – the people who will never complain (as they don't know how to) or who will just quietly die'.[14]

'I am absolutely certain', says Nichole, 'that the stress she endured caused her to give up her fight against her illnesses. Without the stress we would have had a little more precious time.'[13]

How did governments and agencies respond to the life expectancy crisis?

Gregory:	Is there any other point to which you would wish to draw my attention?
Holmes:	To the curious incident of the dog in the night-time.
Gregory:	The dog did nothing in the night-time.
Holmes:	That was the curious incident.

Arthur Conan Doyle, The Adventure of Silver Blaze[1]

Given the unprecedented nature of the life expectancy crisis described in the book thus far, you might reasonably expect there to have been an urgent and comprehensive response from governments, from public health agencies tasked with protecting and improving the health of the public and from statistical agencies whose central role is the monitoring of 'vital events' (including deaths) in the UK. What actually happened is startling, because those with these responsibilities were almost entirely silent.[2] This chapter details this 'curious incident', and explores why the metaphorical 'dog' did not bark.

The challenge of identifying a change in life expectancy trends

With some trends it is possible to know quickly when a change has happened. To do this, you need access to up-to-the-minute data which include precise data points corresponding to short time periods such as days or weeks. Understanding when a trend has changed is much more difficult when the opposite is true: where there are delayed, infrequent and imprecise data points.

Life expectancy data are available only once a year, and a few years of data are required in order to understand the trend.[3] Other deaths data are available – for example, the count of the number of people who die each week – but these are useful only for understanding the short-term effects of things like influenza, heat waves and cold spells.[4] They are *useless for understanding long-term trends* because the baseline which is being compared against keeps changing and resetting. For example, if mortality is increasing, the weekly comparison will be with an increasing number over time, hiding the problem. Life expectancy calculations account for these problems, allowing the real changes in mortality to be isolated.

In the UK, the publication of mortality and life expectancy data is the responsibility of the Office for National Statistics (ONS) (for England and

Wales), the Northern Ireland Statistics and Research Agency (NISRA) and National Records for Scotland (NRS). However, these statistical agencies restrict their role to ensuring that the data are correct (through the publication of national statistics and official statistics), rather than interpreting the data to say *why* mortality and life expectancy trends might be changing. Instead, this interpretation is the role of public health agencies, and in particular their so-called 'observatory' functions. Although some public health agencies also produce national statistics and/or official statistics, they also have a broader role to *explain* trends and inform policy makers and the public. Indeed, the medical leaders of these agencies are duty bound by the General Medical Council (GMC) to make the populations they are responsible for their primary concern, rather than the interests of politicians.

A timeline of events

In Chapters 1–3, we described the changing mortality and life expectancy trends in the UK, and how austerity policies are the most important cause. In this section we discuss how governments, public health agencies and relevant 'think-tanks' reacted to these trends. We argue that silence, misdirection, inaction and, arguably, 'denialism' characterise this response. As already noted, it is only in retrospect that it is possible to know that mortality and life expectancy trends have changed. However, in this chapter we show that the evidence that austerity was causing the trends was already available, and a meaningful response could (and should) have resulted. We also demonstrate that even in late 2023 (at the time of writing), several important institutions continue to deny or downplay the role of austerity.

As we also noted in earlier chapters, the 2007 global financial crash, and the consequent 'Great Recession',[5] led to substantial financial problems for governments around the world. The length and depth of the economic downturn varied across countries, but was severe enough to prompt radical changes in policy by both governments and international financial institutions. In the UK, the initial period of money creation (known as 'quantitative easing') and additional borrowing stopped in June 2010 when the incoming Conservative-Liberal Democrat coalition argued that reducing government borrowing through reduced public spending was a more effective means of stimulating economic growth, leaning on the same 'neoliberal' economic doctrine that we discussed in the previous chapter. And thus, the programme of austerity that we have described throughout this book began.[6,7]

Even before the changes to mortality and life expectancy trends in the UK had occurred, a number of academics had pointed out that both the recession and the austerity policy response were likely to have potential adverse consequences for population health.[8–12] Much of this early research focused on particular causes of death, in particular suicides,[9,11,13–15] in countries such as Greece which (as we described in Chapter 4) had been forced by international financial institutions and the European Union to implement large and widespread public spending cuts.[16] However, some of these early studies were prone to criticism, as they tended to focus on very specific issues in very short time periods (with a lack of clarity on why particular populations, outcomes and comparisons were used), rather than providing a comprehensive, longer-term, overview of changes to the health of the affected populations.[9,17]

Nonetheless, these studies added to the existing mass of evidence on the importance of economic policy (and resulting economic circumstances) for the health of populations,[18–24] and specifically pointed out the potential damaging effects of austerity. And such is the scale of this economic–health evidence that it was well known to those in public health agencies and governments, and to other academics who would write about the mortality changes in the UK a few years later. No one could claim that economic changes were irrelevant to changing mortality trends, nor claim ignorance of that evidence when the changed trends became apparent. And yet this evidence was effectively ignored in so much of the discussion that followed.

Table 5.1 provides a timeline of the key events relevant to the life expectancy trends, and the dates when important parts of the evidence base became available. Reports that deny or downplay the role of austerity are shown in bold type – invariably these are by Public Health England or health think-tanks. The list provides a brief summary of the evidence available to governments and agencies during this unprecedented time of changing life expectancy. It expands upon the table of studies which show a causal relationship between austerity and mortality provided in the Appendix.

The emergence of influenza as the key explanation for the 'mortality spike'

As noted in Chapters 1–3, despite the 'Great Financial Crash' (in 2007/08) and a marked economic downturn, overall life expectancy continued to improve in the UK until around 2012. The precise years when the change happened were able to be confirmed only in hindsight, after enough annual data points for life expectancy had been published.[69,117,118] However, in the early months of 2015 the different teams working in public health agencies across Europe monitoring infectious diseases (in particular, influenza) had noticed higher-than-expected deaths in the weekly mortality data.[31]

The weekly mortality data were being fed into a computer model which compared the crude number of deaths in each week for countries across Europe with the number of deaths in the same week in the previous few years. If the number of deaths was higher than in previous years, this was termed 'excess mortality'. Other data from laboratories on the circulation

Table 5.1: Timeline of research published on the role of economics and austerity, with publication of reports denying austerity as a cause in bold type*

UK austerity starts

2010   • Landmark health inequalities report (Marmot Review) shows importance of economic policy[18]

2011   • Austerity linked to HIV outbreak in Greece[25]

2012   • Austerity linked to worsening health across Europe[17]

2013   • *The body economic: why austerity kills* book published[9]
         • 1 study highlights likely negative impacts of austerity on UK health[26]

2014   • 5 studies link austerity to worse health across Europe[10,27–30]

UK mortality changes first noted in weekly data

2015   • Weekly data show mortality increases in UK[31]
         • *How politics makes us sick: neoliberal epidemics* book published[32]
         • 3 studies investigate austerity impacts on suicide in Europe, 2 show links[13,14,33]
         • Rise in mental health problems in England linked to austerity[34]
         • Austerity linked to rise in food banks in UK[35]
         • Review of evidence from across disciplines on the austerity–health link[11]

2016   • Austerity linked to increased homelessness in England[36]
         • 4 studies link austerity to mortality and health problems in 4 countries[37–40]
         • 3 studies link austerity to mental health problems in UK[41–43]
         • **PHE first suggest influenza as likely cause of the changes[44]**

2017   • First UK study demonstrating austerity as cause of mortality change[45]
         • Study summarising evidence for austerity, and not influenza, as cause of changes in the UK[46]
         • Austerity-related delayed hospital discharges linked to mortality change[47]
         • Qualitative study linking austerity in UK to worse health[48]
         • *The violence of austerity* book published[49]
         • 5 international studies examining links between austerity and health[50–54]
         • **PHE continue to suggest influenza as likely cause[55]**

2018   • Study demonstrates UK social security cuts causing worse mental health[56]
         • 3 studies link worse birth outcomes, health inequalities and mortality to austerity[57–59]
         • 2 qualitative studies link austerity in UK to worse health[60,61]
         • Worsening UK mental health trends linked to austerity[62]
         • 3 studies critique PHE explanations for mortality changes[63–65]
         • **PHE response to critique 'doubles down' on influenza as likely cause[66]**
         • **King's Fund argues against austerity, focusing on specific causes of death[67,68]**
         • **PHE mortality review fails to consider austerity[69]**

2019   • Research commentary discusses why austerity is an important cause[70]
         • *Crippled: austerity and the demonization of disabled people* book published[71]
         • Qualitative study linking austerity in UK to worse health[72]
         • Study links austerity to greater food insecurity[73]

         • 2 large studies of international trends conclude austerity is a cause[74,75]
         • Report commissioned by Health Foundation suggests austerity is a likely cause[76]
         • **Health Foundation says 'limited and inconclusive' evidence for austerity[77]**

Table 5.1: Timeline of research published on the role of economics and austerity, with publication of reports denying austerity as a cause in bold type (continued)

Pandemic starts

2020
- 2 studies show austerity impacts in US[78,79]
- Study demonstrates UK social security cuts causing worsening mental health[80]
- 2 studies show negative impacts of austerity on health internationally[81,82]
- Qualitative study linking austerity in UK to worse health[83]
- Update to the Marmot Review of health inequalities in England concludes austerity is driving changed trends[84]
- Public Health Wales report states austerity is a likely contributor to the changed trends[85]
- **King's Fund/OECD argue against austerity, focusing on specific causes of death[86]**

2021
- Modelling study shows austerity explains mortality change in Scotland[87]
- 2 studies demonstrate austerity causing mortality change in England[88,89]
- 4 studies link austerity to food bank use, worse mental health and drug deaths[90–93]
- Study links austerity to rising childhood obesity[94]
- Study summarises the evidence for austerity causing mortality changes[95]
- Scottish CMO report includes austerity as explanation[96]

Inflation rises

2022
- 10 studies using different methods demonstrate austerity's health and social harms[97–108]
- Study shows local government cuts causally linked to higher nutritional anaemia (a marker of malnutrition)[93]
- Glasgow University/Glasgow Centre for Population Health report concludes austerity is main cause[109]
- **King's Fund argue that the causes of the changed trends remain unclear[110]**

2023
- 3 studies show austerity causing mental health, obesity and mortality problems[111–113]
- Study links austerity period with changed trend in severe mental illness[114]
- Health Foundation report on Scottish trends acknowledges role for austerity but focuses on 'implementation gap' as explanation[115]
- **UK CMOs argue that high mortality can be addressed with CVD interventions[116]**

---

* This is in no way a fully comprehensive list of relevant literature in this area, and there are likely to be other relevant studies that we have missed (in particular, highly relevant qualitative studies).

of influenza virus, and temperature information, were then added into the model to estimate how much of this 'excess mortality' was due to influenza, hot or cold weather, or 'other' causes.[119–121]

The public health teams using these models interpreted the high mortality in early 2015 as being due to influenza.[31,119] This was not unprecedented. Indeed, the models had often previously identified periods of excess mortality in particular countries, and had attributed most of these to excess temperatures (hot or cold), or to influenza. Rarely did the models suggest that the excess was unexplained, or that there was – in the terms of the model – an 'other' cause.[120–123]

By late 2015, the weekly counts of deaths had returned to approximately the levels seen in previous years, leading the higher mortality in the earlier months to be characterised by those in the public health teams monitoring infections as a '*mortality spike*'.[44,119] This implied a short-lived, if severe, cause. By 2015 the comparison of weekly deaths with previous years was also now including years after the trends changed, and so this method of monitoring mortality trends was already underestimating the problem. Nevertheless, when the annual life expectancy statistics were published for 2015 (in August 2016), there was already a strong public health voice which was authoritatively stating that most of the excess mortality could be explained by a particularly severe influenza epidemic (see the 2015 and 2016 rows in Table 5.1).[31,44,119,124]

The next section details whether and how, as the evidence of the true causes began to emerge, public health agencies discharged their *duty* to identify and explain the causes of the changing life expectancy trends, and to advise governments of appropriate responses.

The response of public health agencies

England

Public Health England (PHE), along with the English Chief Medical Officer (CMO), were the key public health advisors to the UK government throughout this time period. It was their advice and reports that were quoted by UK government ministers, and it was their briefings that made their way through civil service channels to the politicians.

As part of a pan-European group monitoring weekly deaths data, the infectious disease team in PHE had been tracking the higher number of deaths in early 2015 and had attributed this to influenza.[31,44,119] In July 2017, PHE published a blog which argued that some of the stalled trends could be explained by population ageing and influenza. Austerity was not mentioned as a possible cause, despite at least 22 research reports and books linking it to worse health having been published by the end of 2016 (see Table 5.1). The only recommended responses were further monitoring of the trends and more research. However, this PHE narrative was by now coming under public attack by academics who were pointing out the inadequacies of the influenza explanation and highlighting the need to look to the economic causes of the trends.[46,64,64,125]

The response of PHE in early 2018 was defensive at best.[66,70] Their explanation for the changed trends continued to focus on the role of influenza, as well as highlighting the contribution of various specific causes of death such as heart disease (but without linking this to any underlying factors that might have caused such specific disease trends to change). Perhaps most notable of all was the lack of urgency or concern that this represented a major public health emergency. For example, by this time life expectancy was now falling rapidly for people living in the most deprived areas, but this did not seem to merit recommendations for a policy response.[126,127] It was as if people dying earlier in poorer areas didn't matter.

Throughout 2018 and 2019 there were regular discussions involving all four of the UK public health agencies, the statistical offices and (for some of the meetings) relevant academics and think-tank members (including the King's Fund and the Health Foundation).[128] Before being sidelined by the arrival of the COVID-19 pandemic, these discussions sought to come up with an agreed understanding of the causes of the changed trends with which to advise ministers and the four UK CMOs. Despite this, there was little agreement on the urgency of the issue, nor of the underlying causes.

At the end of 2018, PHE published their summary of the changes to life expectancy and the evidence for the causes.[69] This was their first substantive report on the trends, and it was subsequently used extensively by UK government ministers to defend their inaction on the trends. It was remarkable in two key aspects. First, there was still no alarm about what was going on: there was nothing about urgency, or the scale of the changed trends, or the need to treat this as a public health emergency.[129,130] Second, it made little attempt to review the evidence of all the likely underlying causes of the changes. Within the main body of the report, 'austerity' was not mentioned once (even though by this point at least 41 separate research studies and books had been published making the link [see Table 5.1]). There was a brief review of the potential role of health and social care funding specifically, but it was argued that the evidence for this was unclear. The report took the approach of 'don't ask, don't tell', ignoring the large body of evidence already demonstrating the role of austerity, and, as a consequence, misdirecting and misleading the public.

The report's conclusion said it all:

> This slowdown is unlikely to be caused by problems with the data or methods of analysis used to monitor the trend. It is not possible, however, to attribute the recent slowdown in improvement to any single cause and it is likely that a number of factors, operating simultaneously, need to be addressed.[69]

There were no recommendations for policy action, and, as the COVID-19 pandemic arrived, attention was diverted elsewhere. PHE was subsequently disbanded, with its health improvement functions taken into the UK government Department of Health's Office for Health Improvement and Disparities' (OHID).

Scotland

In Scotland prior to April 2020, the public health responsibility for understanding and explaining mortality trends was shared across several National Health Service (NHS) agencies, with coordination provided by the Scottish Public Health Observatory (ScotPHO).[131] Similar to the story in England, the initial work and explanations for the stalled life expectancy trends focused on influenza, not least because of the extensive collaboration across the UK nations and continental Europe on health protection matters.[31,123] Despite this slow start, regular meetings were convened to include expertise from across Scotland, with accountability and authority from the Scottish Directors of Public Health (DsPH) group.[133]

In 2017, members of this Scottish group instigated UK-wide discussions in order that coherent public health advice could be communicated to civil servants, CMOs, ministers and the public. Initially, the approach in Scotland was to publish research in the academic literature rather than as institutional reports. These were broadly descriptive in the first instance, investigating the timing, age groups, specific causes of death, international trends and inequalities in the trends. Over time, more research was published by the Scottish team which considered the underlying causes.[103,117,118,126,127,129,134,135] There was greater acceptance of the austerity evidence in Scotland, and team members regularly briefed the press, civil servants, elected politicians, the CMO and leaders of various public sector institutions across Scotland on the causal role austerity was playing, with increasing certainty over time.[96,136]

The Scottish CMO, Professor Gregor Smith, supported by one of us, highlighted the issue of stalled life expectancy trends in his 2020–21 annual report, but hedged his bets on the likely causes:

> while acknowledging that austerity may have contributed toward some excess deaths, [other studies] suggest that there could be other explanations such as the growing complexity of medical conditions in our ageing population, the contribution of decelerating improvements in cardiovascular disease (CVD) mortality, and periodic bad flu seasons.[96]

As a consequence of this hedging of bets, there was no clear call to action to address the stalled trends in the report.

In April 2020, during the first wave of the pandemic, the three national public health functions in Scotland[137] (NHS Health Scotland, ISD [Information Services Division] and HPS [Health Protection Scotland]) were brought together to form a new national health improvement organisation, Public Health Scotland (PHS). As noted in Chapter 3, we published a comprehensive report detailing all of the published evidence for the causes of the stalled trends in 2022. PHS staff had led this work and

PHS had scheduled publication. However, the new senior management (and it should be stressed that this has since changed again) decided that they did not want PHS to publish it because it showed clear evidence of political decision making causing the changed mortality trends. For the PHS management at the time this was too sensitive an issue, despite leadership on the causes of health trends being a core role for the organisation. Instead, it was published jointly by the Glasgow Centre for Population Health and the University of Glasgow, where some of the authors worked.[109]

Wales and Northern Ireland

The public health capacity in Wales and Northern Ireland is less than that of England and Scotland, and the general approach taken in both nations was to collaborate on a pan-UK basis to better understand the trends. Descriptive analyses of the changing trends were undertaken,[138] but there was little or no analysis of the underlying causes.[139] That said, and in stark contrast to England, by 2020 the stalled life expectancy trends in Wales *were* interpreted as being plausibly caused by austerity – using a report[84] by the team at University College London (the Institute for Health Equity, led by Professor Michael Marmot) as supporting evidence: 'as Sir Michael Marmot's recent review highlighted, a link between austerity and worsening health and health inequalities is "entirely plausible"'.[85]

World Health Organisation (WHO)

Remarkably, the international agency with responsibility for health (the WHO) has published nothing on the stalled life expectancy trends. The WHO's Global Health Observatory publishes comparable data across countries, but without interpretation or explanation.

The WHO Director-General's foreword for their landmark publication, *World Health Statistics*, makes fleeting reference to the stalled trends, although none of the specifics around either all-cause mortality or life expectancy trends are mentioned: 'However, even before the COVID-19 pandemic, beginning in 2015, progress against many global health indicators had slowed or stagnated.'[140] As such, unprecedented changes to population health seem to have been completely ignored by the organisation established to monitor and lead on global health trends. The changed life expectancy trends were almost completely overlooked; there was no discussion or interpretation of this important public health emergency. Some of this might be explicable, but not excusable, by the hollowing-out of the WHO's surveillance functions. For example, the WHO 'burden of disease' study, which described mortality and ill-health trends across the world, was discontinued in the face of large-scale funding from the Bill and Melinda Gates Foundation for an alternative study, the 'Global Burden of Disease' (GBD) study. Ironically, despite this massive influx of funding, the GBD studies have also said next to nothing about the stalled life expectancy trends. For example, in relation to the US, they noted only that inequalities have increased and, 'improvements in life expectancy ... between 2010 and 2019 were somewhat less than they had been between 2000 and 2010'.[141]

Think-tanks and academics

Think-tanks are institutions which have non-governmental funding sources and which regularly produce reports to inform policy decisions and public debates. Readers might expect health think-tanks to be free from political constraints and pressure, and to provide a more evidence-informed contribution to debates. Of course, not all think-tanks operate as such, with the infamous 'Tufton Street' lobbyists representing the archetypical example of 'dark money' being used to influence public and political understanding for ideological ends.[142]

Two health think-tanks – the Health Foundation and the King's Fund – have substantial influence in the UK, and have published reports on the causes of the stalled life expectancy trends. In 2019, research commissioned by the Health Foundation from the London School of Economics (LSE) to better understand the issue was published.[76] This report examined a wide range of potential causes and tried to distinguish between the causes of short-term fluctuations and the longer-term trends, concluding that austerity could plausibly be contributing. However, the Health Foundation decided to produce their own report which barely referenced the LSE findings. Instead, the Health Foundation conclusion was much more in line with the PHE 2018 report in that it did not include a role for austerity. Instead the Health Foundation argued that: 'There is no single cause of the slowdown, and no single solution: instead actions must be taken on the wider factors that shape the conditions in which people are born, grow, live, work and age.'[77] Note that this Health Foundation report, published as it was in 2019, came at a time after which *more than 44 studies* linking the changed trends to austerity had been published (see Table 5.1), including many of the higher-quality causal studies (see the Appendix).

In 2022, by which point *more than 59 studies* had been published linking austerity to the changes, the King's Fund, echoing the conclusions of the Health Foundation report, argued that (in England): 'The reasons for the post-2011 slowdown in life expectancy improvements are unclear and have been hotly debated.'[110] Bizarrely, it was argued by the King's Fund in this report that austerity was an unlikely cause because some other European countries who had experienced similar changes to life expectancy '*didn't adopt austerity policies'*,[110] citing Germany and Sweden as examples. In fact, as we have seen in the previous chapter, Germany *did* adopt austerity policies, as did Sweden and almost every high-income country for at least some of the relevant time period.[103] The lack of any definition or measurement of austerity in their report, including any analysis to examine its contribution, completely undermines this assertion. Furthermore, none of the international research that was available at the time of the report was cited (see Table 5.1).[14,74,75] Given this, it is unsurprising that the conclusion the King's Fund draws is uninformative and represents a call for further *inaction*. Instead, it simply highlights which cause-specific mortality trends are responsible for explaining the overall life expectancy figures, while shedding no light on the underlying causes.

The views of the Health Foundation and King's Fund stand in stark contrast to the evidence from the academic literature summarised in Chapter 3 (and partly in Table 5.1), and to the informed views of key academics. For example, in 2020 Professor Michael Marmot (author of key reports on health inequality trends in England[18,84]) was quoted in *The Guardian* as saying:

> Austerity has taken a significant toll on equity and health, and it is likely to continue to do so. If you ask me if that is the reason for the worsening health picture, I'd say it is highly likely that [it] is responsible for the life expectancy flat-lining, people's health deteriorating and the widening of health inequalities.[143]

However, due to the selective use of the evidence by think-tanks and some public health agencies, the views they promoted have added to the perception that the evidence is unclear, and therefore that an urgent policy response has not been required. It has allowed politicians to avoid being held to account for the impacts of their policies.[69,76,109,144,145]

The nature of academia is that researchers generally have substantial autonomy to determine their own research priorities and interests. Unlike public health agencies and governments, there are no statutory duties or responsibilities to research in particular areas, although the availability of research funding will have substantial influence. Throughout this book we have cited numerous researchers whose work has been instrumental in identifying the change in mortality trends, and in investigating the causes of these trends. However, academia is not entirely blameless in all this.

In Chapter 4 we described how, outside of the UK and US, there has been almost no research undertaken to understand why mortality trends have changed. Indeed, in many of these countries there has been only the most basic of descriptive studies undertaken. This might reflect a lack of research leadership, a lack of research autonomy or funding, or insufficient public health research generalists who are interested in broad public health trends rather than specific diseases, specific causes or particular interventions. Well-funded international research collaborations such as the Institute for Health Metrics and Evaluation (IHME) and (as already mentioned) their GBD study, have been found wanting, merely noting increases in some specific causes of mortality and age groups without any consideration of the broader causes.[146]

What is behind the different interpretations of the changed life expectancy trends?

We cannot be certain why people working in public health agencies have had such different interpretations of the evidence and data.[145] However, there are some parallels to how the causes of, and appropriate responses to, health inequalities more generally are differently understood.[147–149] Our own experience of being integral to these austerity discussions has led us to suggest four key reasons for the failure to act, and for the consistent misinterpretation of scale, urgency and causes of the problem.

First, people working in public health agencies frequently come under implicit pressure, and occasionally explicit pressure, to avoid 'embarrassing' or 'undermining' governments (both the UK government and the devolved administrations). This means that causes that relate to policy or funding decisions are frequently under-studied, omitted and downplayed. In their place, politically acceptable causes and solutions are focused upon, whether these are individualised behaviours such as smoking or drinking alcohol, or events seen to be outside the control of governments, such as influenza outbreaks. At best, vague references to the 'social determinants of health' or 'socioeconomic inequalities' are made, as if these are immovable, natural facts of life, and not themselves politically determined.[21] The pressure felt by people in senior positions in public health agencies leads to a form of self-censorship, where they embody an understanding of what 'gets them into trouble' or causes 'raised eyebrows'; as a result, they tailor their advice and contributions accordingly. This leads to an avoidance of difficult questions or inconvenient evidence and – as we said earlier in relation to PHE – a 'don't ask, don't tell' approach. In public health the duty is to put the health of populations first, not to spare the blushes of civil servants or politicians. Where the latter happens, it is therefore a profound dereliction of duty.

In our view, this is a problem that permeates the entire chain of advice from public health professionals, through civil servants and government medical officers, all the way to politicians, such that the latter rarely have to impose any explicit censorship themselves. Instead of 'evidence-based policy', this leads to 'policy-based evidence' – a predominance of evidence that supports the current dominant policy approach, irrespective of its quality.[150,151] As one small example, Professor Michael Marmot recounts how two different reports which synthesised the same evidence on what works to reduce alcohol harms came to opposite conclusions because one was seeking to fit with the existing political approach rather than fairly represent the evidence.[151] It is worth noting that these explicit and implicit pressures may be quite different across the UK devolved administrations, as the public health agencies are accountable to politicians from different political parties, who have different priorities and levels of comfort with the austerity explanation.

Second, people working in public health who do propose political causes for population health trends are often dismissed as 'ideological' or 'idealistic'.[152,153] This form of alienation leads to some individuals, theories and evidence being dismissed without being given serious consideration, despite the overwhelming evidence of the political nature of health inequalities, and of political and economic decisions impacting on population health more generally.[18–20,22,23,78,154–157]

Third, it is clear that wildly different thresholds for evidence quality are used to explain different public health problems. For example, PHE continued to propose population ageing as an important cause of the stalled life expectancy trends up to early 2018, despite simple statistical age adjustments showing that this was not the case.[117] Similarly, the evidence that influenza was an important cause of the changed mortality trends was based on analyses that could not explain longer-term trend changes.[120] The suggestion by others that fewer new treatments for CVD might explain the trends has also been given credence, despite a lack of evidence.[86] Yet, because these were seen to be 'safe' explanations that didn't challenge governments, the very low quality of evidence suggesting these as important explanations was nevertheless accepted. In contrast, explanations that did arise from political decision-making, such as austerity, were completely omitted from analyses of potential causes. This despite, as we have already seen, the existence of a large evidence base that had been produced by multiple, independent research teams, using different methods and datasets, almost all of which were reviewed and approved by other researchers in the field, and all pointing towards the same conclusion (see Table 5.1). This 'low evidence' approach was true of the influential 2018 PHE report,[69] which UK government ministers frequently cited to dismiss suggestions that austerity was a cause, but was also true of important reports from the Health Foundation and King's Fund.[67,77,86]

A clear example of the use of different evidence thresholds arises from our experience of discussions with the Department for Work and Pensions (DWP) on the impacts of their 'welfare reforms' on health. The DWP would frequently cite case studies of individuals who had been 'helped' by the reforms, usually to move into paid employment, as strong evidence that the system was working. Yet, when case studies of individuals harmed by these same reforms were put forward, these would be dismissed as 'anecdotes' and 'isolated examples'.

It has long been recognised that it is more difficult to create high-quality evidence for the kinds of causes we discuss in this book, such as economic policies and 'welfare reforms', because this evidence does not come from 'clinical trials' in which patients are randomly allocated to receive real or fake treatments in order to be sure what the effectiveness of different options is.[158] Yet, for the causes of the stalled life expectancy trends, the evidence for austerity is of a *higher quality* than that for influenza,[109] but influenza has still been given greater prominence in key reports (see Table 5.1).

Finally, it is also clear that many (although not all) of those in leadership and decision-making positions (particularly in the UK government, but also across public health agencies and relevant think-tanks), occupy markedly privileged positions in society. Many have had little direct experience of poverty, discrimination or disadvantage, and have incomes in the top 1 per cent of the population distribution. This inevitably shapes their world-view and priorities.[159] These are positions of power, and provide the ability to set agendas, act as gatekeepers for what is classed as a public health problem and, ultimately, make decisions.[160,161] There are obviously exceptions. Many of our own colleagues use their positions of power and influence to consistently advocate for reducing inequalities, and to prioritise research and work that contributes to a more equal society.

The next section goes on to discuss how elected politicians, and in particular UK government ministers, discussed the changed mortality trends, reflecting the issues of power already noted.

Government and political responses

For those unfamiliar with how government operates, it is important to understand the difference between ministers – the elected politicians[162] who are the ultimate decision-makers and have the power to direct policy – and civil servants, who are the permanent staff who work to support the development and implementation of policy, and who are bound by the civil service code of impartiality. 'Government' is a term that includes both the politicians and civil servants. In this section we focus particularly on the responses of UK government ministers, not least because there has been so little discussion of changed mortality trends in other jurisdictions. The nature of the responses falls into a small number of categories, all characterised by the failure to recognise the urgency and importance of the changes to life expectancy. The responses also reveal a form of denialism of the evidence that austerity is the key cause of the changed trends.[163,164]

Avoiding the question

On several occasions, opposition MPs have asked questions, or used their parliamentary debating time, to hold debates on the issue of changed life expectancy trends in the Westminster Parliament. A frequent and standard response to such questions has been to obfuscate and avoid giving a direct answer. For example, in response to the question, 'What recent assessment has she made of trends in the level of life expectancy?' the minister in question said (and this is the full answer, not a selective quotation):

> Although life expectancy at birth remains the highest it has been, we want everyone to have the same opportunity to have a long, healthy life, whoever they are, wherever they live and whatever their background. We are committed to giving everyone five extra years of healthy life by 2035, and to addressing the needs of areas with the poorest health[165] (Nadine Dorries MP, Parliamentary Under-Secretary of State for Health and Social Care, Conservative, 28 January 2020)

Another example, from October 2022, was in response to a question from Scottish National Party (SNP) MP Alison Thewliss, who asked: 'The Glasgow Centre for Population Health published some research that attributed about 330,000 excess deaths since 2010 to austerity – the Tory austerity by the Minister and his colleagues over the past 12 years – so will he cancel any further cuts, because they cost Scotland and our neighbours far more than we can ever afford?'[166] The government spokesperson replied as follows, completely avoiding the question, and simply engaging in what is often termed '*whataboutery*', whereby other issues are raised to deflect attention from the issue at hand:

> The Scottish Government are of course receiving record levels of funding, and that will continue. The Honourable Member asked about excess deaths. Well, I think the drug death record of the nationalist Government is, frankly, pretty terrible.[166] (Chris Philp, Chief Secretary to the Treasury, Conservative, 12 October 2022)

It is also interesting that this '*whatabout*' response contains no denial that government policies have caused hundreds of thousands of extra deaths.

As can be seen in these examples, ministers frequently 'filibuster' by talking in general terms and using data very selectively (if at all), to avoid addressing the issue. The inability of parliamentarians, and the public, to hold ministers to account for this kind of truth–avoidance is surely a major shortcoming of the current system of democracy in the UK.

Demonisation of people on social security benefits and blaming individuals for the trends

After the election of the Conservative-Liberal Democrat coalition government in May 2010, a concerted effort was made by ministers to reframe the economic challenges of the country. The role of the finance sector in causing the economic downturn and government deficit was downplayed, and instead it was repeatedly argued that moving people off social security benefits should be a key priority to promote economic growth. George Osborne, the Chancellor of the Exchequer at the time, said: 'You cannot tackle Britain's debts without tackling the unreformed welfare system. ... If someone believes that living on benefits is a lifestyle choice, then we need to make them think again' (8 June 2010).[167]

Blaming individual behaviours for health outcomes has a long history, despite the strong evidence that behaviours are heavily influenced and determined by broader social and economic forces, and the evidence that inequalities in health are primarily determined by the extent of inequalities in income, wealth and power within societies.[157] This narrative of blaming individuals was also prominent in the UK government explanation for the stalled life expectancy trends:

> Successive Governments have tried to direct resources to help that group of people, but it is still not working. That leads to the realisation that this is as much about behaviour and leadership as it is about money. ... If we take a lifestyle approach to securing the best possible health outcomes and tackling inequalities, an individual's start in life is the beginning of that. ... Broader public education about the impact of sugar is helping, but there is much more we can do to encourage people to adopt healthier lifestyles.[168] (Jackie Doyle-Price MP, Parliamentary Under-Secretary of State for Health, Conservative, 18 April 2018)

Not only does this misunderstand the causes of the changed trends, it unfairly lays the blame for the changes on those who are not responsible, and simultaneously absolves politicians from responsibility. It is thus both disingenuous and misleading.

Arguments that the evidence of the causes of the stalling is uncertain

On those occasions when ministers have been obliged to address the changed life expectancy trends more directly, a common response has been to argue that the evidence on the causes is uncertain, and as a result there are no clear policy implications:

Public Health England's recent review made it clear that it is not possible to attribute the slowdown to any one cause. It is therefore important to tackle all the causes of the deterioration in life expectancy, which is why the Government will publish a prevention Green Paper later this year.[169] (Stephen Hammond MP, Minister for Health, Conservative, 25 April 2019)

I think it would be premature to draw too many conclusions at this stage about the causes of those [life expectancy trends] and whether this is a long-term trend.[168] (Jackie Doyle-Price MP, Parliamentary Under-Secretary of State for Health, Conservative, 18 April 2018)

The explicit use of the PHE report to make this argument is particularly disappointing, as it provides ministers with a gloss of being informed and in line with public health advice and evidence.

In another example, the fact that life expectancy improvements stalled across different countries was used as an excuse for uncertainty and inaction, as if the causes of the changes could arise only in a single country:

It is important to emphasise that this dip in life expectancy is not unique to the UK. We have seen it elsewhere in Europe. We need to be circumspect about drawing too much by way of conclusion.[168] (Jackie Doyle-Price MP, Parliamentary Under-Secretary of State for Health, Conservative, 18 April 2018)

As we discussed in the previous chapter, the evidence that the stalling has occurred across countries is in fact *a strong indicator that the causes are due to common factors across countries*, of which austerity is the most obvious.[103]

Spurious arguments

Another recurrent feature of the responses of ministers to the changed trends has been the use of spurious arguments. These have taken different forms. One argument used is that the stalling of life expectancy was not a problem because: 'life expectancy cannot be expected to increase forever'[170] (Robert Courts MP, Conservative, 18 April 2018). It is unclear whether this answer is simply misinformed or disingenuous, but, as we have already discussed elsewhere in this book, UK life expectancy is substantially below that of other countries such as Japan, and so to suggest that it could not be expected to increase further is incorrect. Furthermore (as we have again pointed out at length), the areas of the UK which have seen the worst changes – increasing death rates and therefore decreasing life expectancy – are the areas where, even prior to the changes, life expectancy was already nowhere near any kind of 'natural limit'.

Disappointingly, the misleading narrative of the King's Fund reports[67,110] (which claimed that Germany did not implement austerity when in fact they did) was also used to suggest that the stalled trends in Germany meant that austerity could not be an important cause in the UK: 'There has been no austerity in Germany, because the Germans live within their means and run a big budget surplus. They have a trade surplus with China. However, life expectancy is falling in Germany as well.'[171] (Andrew Selous MP, Conservative, 18 April 2018).

In June 2023, at the start of the UK COVID-19 inquiry, the two original architects of the UK austerity policies were asked to account for the health impacts of those policies. George Osborne, Chancellor of the Exchequer back in 2010, said that he 'completely rejects' claims that austerity reduced pandemic preparedness; while David Cameron, the Prime Minster at the time, said, 'it was the right economic policy'. Some public health leaders responded with barely concealed fury:

David Cameron's ignoring of the evidence in his COVID inquiry testimony was irritating. George Osborne's was worse.[172] (Professor Michael Marmot, University College London)

For [George Osborne] to say there is 'no connection whatsoever between austerity and the unequal impact of the pandemic on disadvantaged communities' is quite staggering.[173] (Professor Martin McKee, London School of Hygiene and Tropical Medicine)

Conclusion

Public health agencies, and the professionals who work in them, have a duty to monitor, investigate and explain health and mortality trends. In discharging these duties they are obliged to make their 'patients [or in this case, their populations] their first concern',[174] and to be informed by the best available data and evidence. That public health agencies – most notably PHE and the WHO – did not raise the alarm that austerity policies were causing life expectancy to stop improving overall, and causing it to fall rapidly in the most deprived communities, is a dereliction of duty. It is less of a surprise that the politicians responsible for implementing these policies denied their impacts, but those denials were made easier because of the failure of public health agencies and think-tanks to be led by the evidence, especially by 2022 when the evidence base was so robust.

'Denialism' has been described by researchers working on tobacco control as having six features: suggestion of a research conspiracy; use of fake experts; selective referencing of research; creation of impossible expectations of research; misrepresentation and logical fallacies; and manufacture of doubt.[163,164] It can be argued that at least two of these aspects of denialism are evident in the reports discussing why mortality trends have changed. For example, we have presented evidence for selective referencing (that is, the failure to cite relevant research linking austerity and mortality in important reports, including the causal studies [see Table 5.1 and Appendix]). We have also experienced people making impossible expectations of research on the role of austerity. For mortality trends research it is impossible to undertake the same kind of experimental trials that are undertaken for medicines. However, there are a great number of robust studies which account for important sources of bias and which provide causal evidence for the role of austerity (see the Appendix). These studies are substantially more robust than the models which suggested influenza was causing the trends, yet influential people in PHE and think-tanks continued to prefer the influenza explanation. When challenged, the response was often to demand higher-quality evidence of the role of austerity.

We do not argue that austerity explains 100 per cent of changes in life expectancy trends across all countries and time periods; far from it. Nor do we claim that there are no uncertainties in the evidence (not least about the different nature of austerity across countries). But the evidence is clear that austerity is the most important cause of the changes in trends seen across high-income countries after 2010, including in the UK. We must avoid drifting into denialism about this evidence. There are many potential reasons why the public health dog did not bark about the change in life expectancy trends, and lessons need to be learned if the health of populations is to be protected and enhanced in the future.

Ellen

A recurring theme of this book is the manner in which society (or, more accurately, government) treats the most vulnerable people among us. The disabled. The poor. Those with mental health conditions. And also those with drug-addiction issues.

People with an addiction – a medically classified illness[1] – are extremely vulnerable. Vulnerable to all sorts of harm: harm from the drug they rely on; harm from the absence of the drug they rely on; harm from the environment to which their illness exposes them.

As we discussed in Chapter 3, numbers of drug-related deaths have been increasing across all of the UK since early 2010s but rates have been highest in Scotland by some distance. The reasons for this are well understood (at least by researchers, if not by many politicians) and relate to a complex set of factors. These include, first, an ageing, vulnerable (that word again) generation of drug users who were born in the 1960s and 1970s in the poorest parts of the country, who were particularly affected by the politics and economic conditions of the 1980s (accelerated deindustrialisation, poverty and inequality), and who have since experienced multiple health conditions as they have become older. Second, the price and affordability of drugs: relatively speaking, street drugs are much cheaper now than they were several decades ago. Third, the different types of drugs on the market, some of which have been implicated in particular 'spikes' of drug deaths in recent years. Fourth, the availability of drugs, including sophisticated drug supply networks. And last but not least (as we discussed in Chapter 3), austerity.[2–5]

In many ways, Ellen's story is, sadly, very typical of many people with severe drug-addiction issues in Scotland, and indeed the UK. Born in a poor part of one of Scotland's main cities, Ellen had faced all sorts of difficulties in early life, and by the time she came into contact with social work services in the city she had a serious opiate-addiction problem. By the early 2010s – the start of the period that this book focuses on – she was in her late 20s and, by then, a long-term, chronic, substance user. She also had three young children. She had an illness and needed help; her children, victims of circumstance, also needed help. But austerity, introduced by the UK government in 2010, did not help; it did the opposite. It provided more of the harm to which Ellen was vulnerable.

At the time, Ellen, and others like her who were struggling to cope with their addiction issues, probably thought that life could not become any more challenging. Little did they know what lay around the corner. The early 2010s marked the start of a serious downward spiral for many. A 'perfect storm' of cuts to funding, reorganisation of services in the city and, especially, changes to the social security benefits on which so many people with addiction issues rely, had a devastating impact. With either less money (because of the social security changes) or no money at all (because of increased benefit 'sanctions'), individuals had to rely more and more on social workers for help. Staff at the time recall increasingly desperate phone calls from clients seeking various forms of assistance. Many social workers spent long hours trying to help clients actually feed and clothe themselves and their families by sourcing food from food banks, and clothes from wherever they could. The reorganisation of services didn't help: it meant that case workers (who, importantly, had forged relationships with clients and were therefore familiar with their lives, needs and broad circumstances) were changed. Funding cuts meant that there were less resources with which to help clients; furthermore, social workers were now having to juggle unmanageable caseloads of 50 or 60 (or, in extreme cases, over 100) clients each.

Surviving on a reduced income (or on no income at all) is obviously hard enough for most people. But for people with an addiction which needs to be satisfied, it's almost impossible. Many – especially those who lived on their own – did precisely that with what little income they could obtain: they fed their habit, and other activities like eating became less important.

Ellen's situation was more challenging yet, as she also had three young children to look after. That meant extra pressure and extra responsibilities. It would be a lie to say that Ellen's situation prior to the implementation of austerity policies was in any way a good one. It was not. However, she was at least – to a degree – able to manage her finances reasonably adequately. She received various social security payments that were helpfully spaced out over the course of each month: income support was provided fortnightly; child benefit and child tax credit at different, regular intervals. In the chaotic circumstances of someone with serious addiction issues, the regularity of those payments over each four-week period is really important. However, key features of the UK government's 'welfare reforms' that were described in Chapter 3 brought all that to a shuddering halt. With three children, the two-child benefits cap reduced Ellen's (and her family's) overall income considerably. Worse, the combining of all benefits into the new Universal Credit payment meant, first, an initial stop to all money (because of the astonishing five- to six-week delay described in the earlier chapter); and then, second, only one payment was received every four weeks (albeit that this was later changed to fortnightly). The problems associated with providing one month's worth of money in a single sum to someone in Ellen's vulnerable circumstances are not hard to fathom. On top of all that, other changes to the system, including lowering the age of children at which their mothers had to prove their work-seeking credentials, catapulted Ellen into the world of threatened 'sanctions' and yet more financial loss and uncertainty. A spiral of even greater misery ensued.

Her case worker describes in detail the devastating impact all this had on Ellen's mental health, on her mood. How could Ellen possibly cope? The answer was not a good one. Her response – her 'coping mechanism' – was to change her drug use, from opiates to benzodiazepines (sedative medication): 'benzos', for short. In part, this was because they were more affordable; but also because the 'numbness' they provided helped her to deal with the circumstances that were spiralling out of control. A cheaper hit to block out the financial reality. However, regular use of, and reliance on, 'benzos' is clearly not without consequences: the impact on both Ellen and her children was acute. The need to feed her addiction in this way to block out the pain led to greater neglect of her children, and they were soon placed on the child protection register. In subsequent years, they would be removed from Ellen completely.

This story does not come with what anyone would describe as a happy ending. Today Ellen is still a substance user, and still a client of social work services in the city. She no longer has any contact with her children. When her mum died, the last vestige of family support disappeared. Yet she is alive. And her children are in a much better place – both literally and figuratively. It would clearly be ridiculous to suggest that Ellen has been 'lucky'. Yet we can certainly say that other substance users in the city have been even less lucky. Ellen's story is all too familiar to people who work in social services in Scotland and the UK; hers is not in any way an extreme case. A great many people numbed the pain of their circumstances – circumstances which, almost unbelievably, austerity policies had managed to make even worse – to the ultimate extent. In the words of another drugs worker we quoted in Chapter 3, people sought 'oblivion' to escape. Between 2010 (when austerity was introduced) and 2021, drug-related death rates in Scotland increased by 142 per cent: in that period 10,435 people died from drug-related causes.[6,7]

6

What else is relevant for understanding the changed life expectancy trends?

Omnishambles.

Malcolm Tucker, BBC's 'The Thick of it'[1]

So far in this book we have focused on how government austerity policies have caused changes to mortality and life expectancy trends in the UK (as well as in many other countries). Austerity policies are undoubtedly the most important factor in explaining the trends. However, there are three other relevant influences that need to be included if we are to have a comprehensive and up-to-date explanation. First are the increases in obesity due to the creation of so-called 'obesogenic environments'. Second are the direct and indirect impacts of the COVID-19 pandemic in 2020 and 2021, especially. And third are the effects of the rapid rise in inflation from 2022 onwards.[2–7] These are discussed separately in more detail in the following sections, but they all interact with one another and with the austerity policies discussed in previous chapters, and should not therefore be considered in isolation from one another. Arguably, the sequence of rising obesity, austerity, the pandemic, followed by the 'costs of living crisis', is best described as a modern-day *'omnishambles'*[1] for mortality trends.

Obesity and the 'obesogenic environment'

Increasing obesity

When people are too heavy it increases their risk of experiencing a wide range of illnesses, as well as early death.[8] There are different ways to measure obesity, but the most appropriate for tracking trends in a population is the Body Mass Index (BMI). Calculated from people's heights and weights,[9] it is a way of estimating whether individuals are an appropriate weight, although it has limitations.[10] The 'healthy' level of BMI is usually defined as between 20 and 25, overweight as 25–30, and obesity as any value over 30. For every five-point increase in the BMI scale, the risk of mortality in European and North American populations has been shown to increase by 39 per cent.[8]

In most rich countries obesity levels have been increasing since the 1990s.[11,12] In 1991 around a fifth of men and a quarter of women living in the US were obese (Figure 6.1). Over the subsequent three decades this has

Figure 6.1: Obesity trends* in the US,[18] England[19] and Scotland[19]

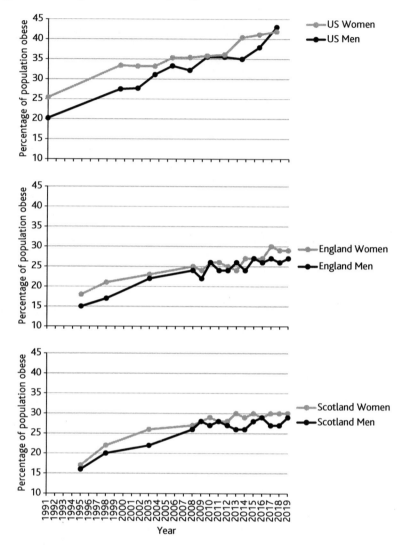

* The US data are for adults aged 20+ years and are age adjusted. For Scotland and England, the data are for the population aged 16+ years, except in 1995 (16–64 years) and 1998 (16–74 years).

increased to around 43 per cent – not far off half of the whole population. The situation in England and Scotland is similar, but less extreme. In the mid-1990s, 15–18 per cent of people were obese, increasing to 27–30 per cent by 2019 (Figure 6.1). Across the US, England and Scotland, the percentage of the population who are obese has tended to be higher for women than men.

In the distant past, being heavy was a marker of wealth and status because it indicated that you could afford to eat rich foods and that you did not need to engage in long hours of manual labour.[13] This form of status was exemplified by the symbolism of the 'big man' in some cultures.[13] This is no longer the case. In rich countries obesity is now much more common in more disadvantaged groups, with stark inequalities in who is most affected.[13–16] This is also increasingly the case in poorer countries.[17]

The causes of increasing obesity

For individuals, becoming too heavy is almost always a consequence of eating too many calories compared to the energy used up through physical activity. There are exceptions to this for some individual health conditions, but these are uncommon. However, to explain why obesity is increasing, it is essential to move beyond individual decisions and behaviours. Obesity has increased across countries because societies as a whole have become more '*obesogenic*': where physical, economic, policy, social and cultural factors interact to promote obesity.[12,20] This means that it has become much more difficult to stay a healthy weight because too many of the influences around us are encouraging weight gain.

The physical environments in which we live have radically changed over recent decades. More roads have been built, and existing roads have been widened and extended. More people have access to cars and use them more often. More workplaces, shops, leisure facilities and houses have been built outside or on the edge of existing towns and cities, and often at motorway junctions.[12,21] This has made it a much easier choice to use cars to get around, and made it more difficult to walk, cycle or use public transport. For example, between 1966 and 2011 in Scotland, the percentage of journeys to work by car increased from 21 per cent to 70 per cent, whilst the percentage for walking to work fell from 24 per cent to 11 per cent, and the percentage for using the bus fell from 43 per cent to 11 per cent.[22]

There has been some pushback against the trend towards more car use. In some cities there have been attempts to reduce the space given over to cars, and to increase that dedicated to cycling and walking.[23] Policies like these, as well as the congestion caused by the increase in car travel, have provided some counterbalance to the overall trends. Nevertheless, our urban environments have radically been redesigned in favour of car travel and privatised space, and with them our physical activity habits.[12]

Workplaces are also unrecognisable from the early 1980s. Many of the jobs which involved physical labour have gone, with the rise in tools, machines and automation. It is much more common now to have a workplace consisting of a chair, desk and computer, and requiring minimal physical exertion. In the past, we would get most of our exercise from our work and from commuting to and from work. Now, most people who get exercise do so as part of leisure activities in the evenings and at weekends. Of course none of this is distributed across populations evenly. Manual work, such as social care or refuse collection, still exists, but tends to be low paid and undervalued. But the general trend is towards a world where work involves staring at a screen for eight hours a day.[24]

Even at home the manual labour of the past has reduced radically. Electric vacuum cleaners, automatic washing machines, food mixers and powered lawnmowers have all reduced the energy we have to spend. It is now almost unheard of for us to have to get out of our chair to change the television channel (for younger readers, television remote controls are a relatively recent invention – in the past you had to get out of your chair, walk over to the television and manually push a button!). Home entertainment has expanded exponentially, with hundreds of television stations, streaming services and internet options. All of which makes it more likely that we will sit in front of the 'box' (or another screen) in our leisure time.

Physical activity patterns for children are dramatically different from the past.[25–28] It is now uncommon to see children playing games together in the streets. When we were growing up, the streets and muddy grass around our homes were alive with mass football games every evening, energetic games of hide–and–seek, skipping, and chases. Instead, play has now become passive, more solitary, and is much more likely to involve games consoles. Where physical activity does happen, it is more likely to be structured, supervised and to involve parents driving children to sports clubs. Many things are behind these changes – the rise in technology (more on which later in this chapter), increased fear of unsupervised play, increased traffic on the roads and urban sprawl (leading to children and young people living further away from one another).[25–28]

On the other side of the obesity equation, our food system has also radically changed. Up until 2022 and the cost-of-living crisis, food had steadily become more and more affordable.[12] Eating out and take-away food had become accessible to more of the population. Within the home, pre–prepared 'ready meals' and highly processed foods have become much more common. Time pressures and increased availability of other leisure pursuits have created a need for more convenient food sources that take less time and effort to prepare, and which can fit into our busy lives. This has vastly reduced home cooking for day-to-day meals.

Sugar, salt and fat have been added to our diets by food companies to make foods more attractive and tastier, and to keep them from spoiling. We are more likely to have more space available to keep foods frozen or refrigerated. We are incessantly subject to advertisements which invoke us to consume more food, and to treat ourselves. Our children are prompted to pester us for sugary snacks – sometimes masquerading as breakfast cereals or 'energy boosters'. Caffeine is added to some products to make sure that we come back for more. Simultaneously, we are told to eat healthily, eat five (or seven) fruits and vegetables a day and to keep our weight at a healthy level. The contradictions are everywhere.[12]

Food is big business, and the food industry's primary concern is not our health.[29,30] In the competition for market share, marketing is essential for companies to increase profits. But this means that more of us are induced to eat more than is healthy for us. Food companies make their products more convenient, sweeter, fattier and tastier.[30] Mass production makes these pre-prepared foods cheaper, with home cooking becoming increasingly an option only for those who have time, money, expertise and kitchen facilities.

The array of changes that have made societies obesogenic are tied into the wider economic and social policy changes seen across many rich countries since the 1980s that we discussed in Chapter 4. For example, the opening up of markets and deregulation that we described extends to the food industry, urban planning and transport.[12,20,31-34] The rise in out-of-town shopping centres, motorways and new roads has been in pursuit of economic growth and profit. The food industry has become just another market in which multinational companies can make profits and can promote maximum consumption.[29,30] Technological developments, including games consoles and smartphones, have facilitated a whole new market: our attention.[35,36] Whether through new smartphone apps and games, social media sites or streaming of videos, our attention is being sold to advertisers, inciting us to consume more while keeping us inactive.[37] Of course, it may not all be bad, with apps encouraging us to take more steps, or to share and compete in running and cycling challenges. But the net impact of globalisation and the ever-greater incursion of neoliberal markets into our lives has been the underlying driver of the obesity epidemic.[12,29-31,34]

It is no wonder that obesity has increased in this context.

How much of the stalled life expectancy trends does obesity explain?

Given that carrying extra weight increases the risk of mortality, and given that there has been an increase in the percentage of people in most richer countries who are obese, it is no surprise that obesity might be playing a role in the stagnating life expectancy trends. Indeed, it was suggested many years ago that increases in obesity could stop improvements in life expectancy.[11,12]

As we discussed briefly in Chapter 3, to understand the extent to which obesity might have contributed to the changed trends, we used an epidemiological technique which compares mortality rates in the population who are obese and those who are not. We then applied this difference in risk of mortality to the number of people in Scotland and England who had become obese in the relevant time period. This allowed us to estimate how much of the stalled trend was potentially due to obesity. The estimate of the contribution of obesity is not exclusive (that is, it does not discount the contribution of other factors, including those which might have made obesity more common, such as changes to the food system, our physical environments and the economy).[38]

As discussed in Chapter 3, there are many uncertainties in these estimates (as was made clear in the published scientific research paper), relating to the underlying data on the number of people who are obese, the quality of the evidence linking obesity to mortality and the assumptions we had to make in our modelling.

As also outlined in Chapter 3, in Scotland obesity was estimated to have contributed approximately 10 per cent of the stalled trends for men and around 14 per cent for women; in England the figures were higher, at 20 per cent for men and 35 per cent for women.[19] These percentages are more likely to be overestimates than underestimates, given the ways in which biases might have affected the data we used.[19] Our estimates of what the mortality trends would have been in 2016–19, had obesity stayed at the level it was at in 1995, are shown for Scotland in Figure 6.2 and for England in Figure 6.3. The black dots represent the actual mortality rates in each year; the gray dots represent what the mortality rate might have been if obesity levels had not increased. Thus, the figures demonstrate that although the change in trends would not have been quite as bad as they actually have been, the impact of other factors (that is, austerity) is clearly much greater (especially in Scotland).

Although there has been no equivalent study for the declining life expectancy trends in the US, as mentioned in Chapter 4, it has been estimated that 55 per cent of the difference in life expectancy between the US and other rich countries can be explained by higher levels of obesity in the US.[39] No comparable estimates are available for other countries, but we know that obesity has increased across most rich countries, and so it is highly likely that obesity is making a similar contribution elsewhere. As Figure 6.1 makes clear, the level of obesity and the rapid increase in the US is substantially larger than in the UK, and so it may be making a greater contribution there. This more rapid rise in the US is no surprise, given that the introduction of neoliberalism, including all of the commensurate changes to food, travel and urban planning, has been implemented more vigorously there.

What impact will obesity have in the future?

Between 2010 and 2017, it looked as if the upward trends in obesity might be levelling off in England and Scotland, mirroring an earlier levelling-off in the 2000s in the US (Figure 6.1). More recently, obesity has been increasing again. Collecting survey data on the percentage of people who are obese has become more difficult since around 2010. The proportion of people who agree to take part in these health surveys has been declining, making

Figure 6.2: Comparison of the actual mortality trends in Scotland in 1991–2019 with the estimated trends, had obesity not increased after 1995[19]

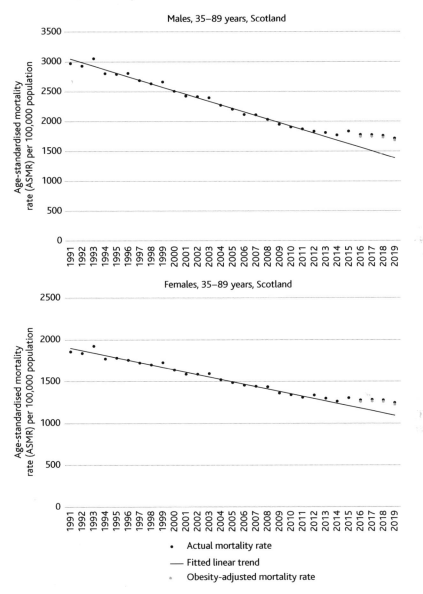

the samples of people who do respond less representative of the population overall.[40] We are therefore much less certain now about the population trends in obesity than we have been in the past.

One of the reasons why obesity increased over the period shown in Figure 6.1 was that food and car travel had become more affordable. However, austerity policies have restricted people's incomes, especially for poorer

Figure 6.3: Comparison of the actual mortality trends in England in 1991–2019 with the estimated trends, had obesity not increased after 1995[19]

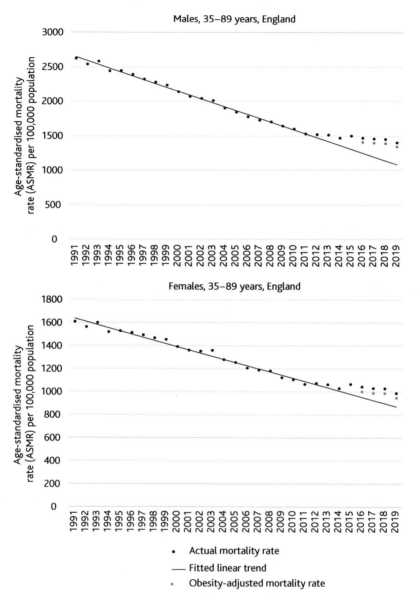

groups. This may be partly why the rate of increase in obesity has slowed in recent years. The rise in inflation from 2022 (discussed in more detail later) might have a similar effect. If obesity increases again in the future, this is highly likely to contribute further to stalling life expectancy. We are also likely to see further negative impacts of the increases in obesity that have already occurred, but which aren't yet evident from the health statistics. However, although increased obesity is likely to have contributed to the changed mortality trends, the scale of impact is relatively small. As mentioned in Chapter 3, what our estimates show is that in England at least 65–80 per cent, and in Scotland at least 86–90 per cent, is *not* related to obesity.[19]

COVID-19

In January 2020, the World Health Organisation (WHO) published a notification of a cluster of pneumonia cases in Wuhan, China.[41] This was the start of a global pandemic which not only caused over 3 million deaths in 2020 alone,[42] but which led to widespread disruption to the everyday lives of people across the world.

The pandemic impacted on the health of populations in a number of ways.[3] First, there were the direct impacts of the virus itself, leading to death, illness and long-term health problems for many. Second, there were the impacts of disruption to the delivery of healthcare services. Third, health was affected as a secondary consequence of the various lockdown measures introduced to reduce the spread of the virus and to give time for vaccinations to be produced to protect people who were exposed. Each of these is discussed in turn in the following sections, highlighting how these have further compounded the already stagnating, or worsening, life expectancy trends.[7]

The direct impacts of COVID-19 infection

Differential COVID-19 exposure

The COVID-19 virus spreads primarily through the air, moving between people as they cough, sneeze and breathe.[43] The risk of being exposed to the virus therefore depends on how many other people you come into contact with, particularly in enclosed and crowded spaces, and where there is a higher likelihood of other people carrying the infection.[43] This put some people at much higher risk than others.[3,44–47] People living and working in shared accommodation (for example, care homes for the elderly or children's care homes) were at risk because of the number of people in the same space with whom they shared facilities. People who worked in hospitals were similarly at high risk – exacerbated by the high likelihood of people they were caring for being infected. Public transport workers, and people who had to use public transport to travel to essential jobs, were also more likely to be exposed to the virus.[44]

We found out during the pandemic that the *essential workers* in our societies also tended to be the *lowest paid and least respected*. Care workers, refuse collectors, delivery drivers, postal workers, people working in food production, as well as healthcare workers and teachers, were all recognised by the media and politicians, if only briefly, as the workers upon whom we all relied.[48] This meant that many of our lowest-paid workers were much more likely to be exposed to the virus, especially in the early phases of the pandemic. Of course, the bad behaviour among political leaders and some more privileged groups, including the UK Prime Minister and his allies, did lead to some other social groups being exposed unnecessarily, putting additional pressure on health services.[49] However, it was predominantly poorer populations who were most impacted.

Even within those groups designated as essential workers, access to personal protective equipment (PPE) – the masks, gowns, gloves and glasses that reduced the transmission of the virus from person to person – was unevenly distributed. All too often, lower-paid workers who still had high levels of exposure (such as social care staff) did not have the same access as better-paid workers who had lower exposure.[44]

People's living arrangements also varied dramatically. Larger families, and especially families with insufficient indoor space, with shared bedrooms and living areas, were at much higher risk of transmitting the virus between them. Poorer households were less likely to have gardens and access to nearby green spaces to exercise, leading to more time spent indoors and greater exposure. Isolation of people who were infected was much more difficult in some households than others. 'Blended families' with shared care arrangements for children across different households were also at higher risk, as this created additional pathways for the virus to spread. Again, all of this meant that the risk of exposure to the virus was much higher among those with less resources.[3,44-46]

How governments responded to the pandemic varied across countries. Some governments (for example, in New Zealand) introduced stringent lockdown measures for prolonged periods of time. Others, like the UK, had a more periodic approach, alternating periods of strict lockdown with times where people were encouraged to go out and socialise (for example, through the now infamous 'Eat Out to Help Out' scheme). The effectiveness of government measures made a big difference to how much virus was circulating within countries at different times through the pandemic. This meant that each individual's risk of exposure depended not only on their own behaviours but also on the effectiveness of the government measures that had been put in place.[50,51]

Differential vulnerability to COVID-19

For the same level of exposure to the virus, there were marked differences in how likely this was to cause severe illness and death across groups. Age is the single most important factor that increases the risk of death in someone exposed to COVID-19.[52] This led to policies being put in place to 'shelter' or 'shield' elderly people and those with weaker immune systems from virus exposure, in order to reduce the mortality impacts of the pandemic. This had other negative consequences on people's lives, such as increased social isolation, that are discussed further in the following paragraphs.

People with existing chronic diseases, especially respiratory conditions, were also at much higher risk of death if they caught the virus.[44,52] Chronic diseases are much more common in poorer communities, meaning that the risk of death, even with the same level of exposure to the virus, was unequal.[44] Across countries, the burden of chronic disease is also unequally distributed, with higher rates of chronic disease estimated in countries like the US and UK than in many other rich countries.[53] Obesity was also found to be an important cause of higher mortality from COVID-19.[54]

The increase in obesity across richer countries since the 1980s, as well as the increase in other chronic health conditions, made populations more *vulnerable* to the impacts of the pandemic when it arrived. Had the pandemic hit when the population was healthier, with less obesity and chronic disease, and in a context where public services hadn't been eroded by austerity, the consequences would have been very different: less people would have died needlessly.[44–46]

The effects of disruption to healthcare services

As the pandemic hit, urgent changes were made to how healthcare services were provided. There was concern at the start of the pandemic that hospital beds would need to be made available for people acutely sick with COVID-19. To prepare for this, routine operations were postponed and patients were moved quickly out of hospitals wherever possible. A range of measures were put in place to reduce overcrowding within healthcare settings, and staff had to change their PPE between patients to avoid cross-contamination and virus spread. This meant that it took longer to assess and treat each patient, whether that was in primary care or in hospital.

The number of people turning up at hospital for treatment for non-COVID-19 conditions dramatically decreased during the early phases of the pandemic,[7] on average by about a third across countries.[55]

There are three possible reasons for this. First, and most obviously, service access was restricted, operations were cancelled and priority was given to emergencies and COVID-19 cases.[56] The expected impact of this is an increase in chronic ill-health, as people missed out on the healthcare that would have benefited them. This meant people living for longer with arthritic joints and cataracts, or going for longer without a diagnosis for unknown conditions. For those people who did attend hospital as an emergency, there is evidence that services were becoming overwhelmed and that the quality of care had deteriorated.[57]

Second, the need for some healthcare might have declined during the pandemic. For example, as most contact sports were outlawed for long periods, a decline in related injuries and fractures might have been expected. The move towards working at home for those who were able to do so also meant less traffic on the roads, resulting in fewer road traffic injuries.[3,58] On the other hand, the pandemic might have increased the need for healthcare for some groups, perhaps due to the increased stress for some workers (for example, in health and social care) or due to the stresses from confinement to the home.[3]

Third, and most importantly, there is evidence that there was a marked decrease in the number of people contacting health services who still needed them. This may have been an unintended consequence of government messaging which tried to reduce the number of people turning up to healthcare services unnecessarily. However, it seems that many people who didn't turn up did actually need care. The number of people diagnosed with cancer dramatically decreased, as did the number of people presenting with acute heart attacks.[7,55,56] The mortality rates from non–COVID-19 conditions increased.[59-62]

The effects of lockdown measures

In addition to the direct impacts of the virus, and the consequences of changes to healthcare delivery, the pandemic is also likely to have had marked impacts as an unintended consequence of the lockdown measures put in place to slow the spread of the virus. This is not to say that the overall mortality impact of the pandemic would have been lower had lockdown measures not been introduced,[51] but it is clear that these have had marked and long-lasting health consequences.[3,7,63]

'Lockdown' is being used here as shorthand for a wide range of different policy interventions introduced across countries during the pandemic. Lockdown isn't one thing, but there are certain common features and impacts that are important. People were asked to stay at home more frequently, which for many people meant loneliness, decreased physical activity, over-consumption of alcohol and food and no escape from abusive relationships.[63] For some other people, particularly those who already had large, comfortable houses with gardens, who perhaps were furloughed and therefore had more time while maintaining an income, and who lived in a household with other supportive people, it could have been a much more enjoyable experience. Social media abounded with stories of people writing books, learning new languages, taking up new creative arts and creating 'home gyms'. This was not the reality for most people, however, and there were profoundly unequal experiences across the population.[3,7,44-46,63]

The worst economic consequences of closing down non-essential businesses were mitigated by the furlough scheme, which provided a source of income for workers who were not allowed to continue to work. Furthermore, social security benefits were temporarily increased in some countries (for example, Universal Credit was increased in the UK by £20 per week). Despite these policies, some workers and businesses lost substantial amounts of income for a prolonged period of time, with some sectors such as hospitality particularly badly affected. The economic pressures people faced during the early phases of the pandemic were mixed. Some costs such as rail and bus travel reduced for some people who could work at home. Childcare costs often decreased as well, but many parents had to juggle home-working, online education and childcare. Other costs increased, such as the cost of fuel to keep houses warm during the day.[3,7,44–46,63]

The changes to the use of transport during the pandemic had mixed impacts on health.[3,7,44–46] Less car travel reduced air pollution (albeit that this was counterbalanced by increased emissions from home heating) and traffic injuries.[63] In many cities infrastructure to support cycling (for example, segregated cycle lanes) was rapidly introduced to make active travel a more attractive option for people, partly to reduce the number of people using public transport and the risks of virus spread. This had the potential to contribute to a longer-term shift in the forms of transport people use towards much healthier modes.[32] However, the extent to which the new infrastructure has been retained and the changes in transport choices have been maintained, has been limited.[63]

Disruption to education, from pre-school all the way through to adult education, had particularly important impacts during the pandemic.[3,7,44–46,63] Education is a very important determinant of health, and, given that there are known critical periods in child development, there was a particular worry that disruption could cause impacts that could not be repaired later on. The extent to which people (both school children and adult learners) engaged with online lessons varied, depending on the technologies available (computers, phones, internet), whether there were quiet spaces at home to work and whether or not there was supportive family around. Even when classes returned to school (and colleges and universities), there were frequently restrictions on what could be done, with physical distancing measures remaining in place and free play (for children) discouraged. As a consequence, both socialisation and formal learning were likely to have been substantially disrupted for a prolonged time period.[63]

The long reach of the COVID-19 pandemic

The pandemic has had substantial, unequal and long-lasting impacts on health, most of them negative.[63] As we've shown in some of the figures in this book, mortality rates increased in the peak COVID years of 2020 and 2021, and failed to improve in 2022 (the latest data available at the time of writing). The longer-term impacts of the pandemic are many. 'Long-COVID', the viral syndrome that has impacted on a substantial proportion of people who were infected, has caused disability and lasting ill-health. The consequences of missed education and socialisation could be seen for decades to come, both in health and in broader social outcomes. And the economic consequences are not only borne by the workers and business who lost income during the pandemic, but have also influenced the economic policy decisions taken by governments following the pandemic. The money paid out during the pandemic in the form of furlough, the increased social security payments and the lost tax revenues have meant that the UK government (and others around the world) have much higher debts now than before the pandemic. If there is further adherence to the neoliberal austerity mantra that government debts and deficits have to be brought down by reduced public spending on services, this likely means another round of austerity, with all the health consequences this will bring.[2,62,64]

There is no doubt that the decline in life expectancy seen across countries in 2020, and to a degree in 2021, was substantially due to the direct impacts of the COVID-19 virus causing infection and death. However, even in 2020 and 2021, the wider impacts of the control measures put in place to reduce the spread of the virus were having substantial health consequences, and most of those were negative. The healthcare that people didn't get when they needed it has caused premature deaths and greater ill-health. The lockdown measures disrupted lives and have had widespread and unequal impacts on all aspects of life and, with that, on people's health. The health consequences of the pandemic are still with us, and are likely to be with us for many years to come. However, the impacts of this pandemic have been much worse than they needed to be. Notwithstanding the mistakes of government in implementing control measures for the virus,[47,49] we were much more vulnerable to the pandemic because of the austerity measures that had been introduced in the years before.[65] The consequences were worse because our obesity rates were higher. The austerity years in the run-up to the pandemic left our public services threadbare and stretched, poverty rising and life expectancy trends in decline for the people living in the poorest areas across the UK. And this is now being compounded by inflation – the final act of the omnishambles[1], which we discuss next.

Inflation

Background to increasing prices

As governments lifted lockdown restrictions, the demand for goods and services in the economy increased quickly. This extra demand outstripped supply because of the backlogs in production caused by the pandemic restrictions. When Russia launched its full-scale invasion of Ukraine in February 2022, this reduced the supply of Ukrainian exports, including much of the global supply of cereal crops. The war, and the resulting trade sanctions on Russia, drove up global oil and gas prices. These pressures rapidly increased prices, especially of fuel and food, generating a cost-of-living crisis.[4,6]

Increasing prices of goods and services need not be a problem if people's incomes are increasing at the same rate. Difficulties arise, as they have from 2022, when prices increase faster than incomes. Workers who are well organised by trade unions, and workers who have powerful negotiating positions (for example, by being in short supply), can respond to inflation by bargaining for (that is, negotiating) higher wages. Sometimes this bargaining can involve taking industrial action, including strike action. Other population groups have less power. Pensioners usually have fixed incomes which are determined by governments (in relation to state pensions) and the (usually fixed) value of any private or occupational pensions they have. However, lots of people (for example, those in precarious jobs) don't have these luxuries, and have been the victims of this rampant inflation.

How unequally has inflation been felt?

In the UK in 2020/21, the average household spent £415 per week on all goods and services.[5] On average, this included £22 on electricity and gas and £69 on food and (non-alcoholic) drinks.[5] However, in the poorest fifth of areas, that household food bill accounted for 20 per cent of total income, compared to only 15 per cent of household income in the richest fifth of areas.[5] Similarly, 9 per cent of household incomes in the poorest areas was spent electricity and gas, as compared to only 4 per cent in the richest areas.[5] This meant that when the prices of food and fuel increased quickly during 2022, the impact was much greater on the budgets of those already struggling.[5]

The UK government introduced a series of policies to subsidise the increases in costs in 2022. The level of support reduced the impacts of inflation and made a bigger difference to the incomes of people living in poorer areas.[5] Nevertheless, the inflation impact after accounting for these policies was equivalent to a 13 per cent rise in prices for the population overall, varying from 16 per cent in the poorest fifth of areas to 12 per cent in the richest fifth.[5]

What has the impact of inflation on mortality been?

It is possible to estimate the impacts of changes in income on mortality in Scotland using a model developed by NHS Health Scotland (now Public Health Scotland).[66,67] This was adapted to consider the impacts of increased inflation on mortality and life expectancy in Scotland in 2022. Reflecting the discussion in Chapter 3 (and in other parts of this book) of the link between income and health (and therefore mortality), it estimated that, as a result of the increases, mortality rates for people aged under 75 years would rise by 6 per cent. However, the impacts were bigger in the poorest areas, with an estimated 8 per cent increase in mortality rates, as compared to only 2 per cent in the richest areas.[5] As a result, inflation seems likely to have exacerbated the austerity-induced changes in mortality trends, and the direct and indirect impacts of the pandemic, creating a 'perfect storm' of exposure to health–damaging effects.[7,65]

These estimated impacts of inflation on mortality relate to 2022 only. Our analysis took account of various measures put in place by the UK government to reduce the impact of rising energy prices – including the Energy Price Guarantee and Cost of Living Support. Had these not been put in place, we estimate that the increases in mortality would have been much greater. It is difficult to predict at the time of writing what will happen to inflation and incomes in the future. Armed conflicts continue to occur across the world, and these generally cause increases in oil and gas prices, feeding inflation. However, some groups of workers have managed to bargain for higher wages, and this will reduce the impacts of inflation for people in work. In the UK, most benefits were increased in line with inflation for 2022 and 2023, but it is unclear if this will be repeated if inflation remains high. The experiences of inflation, government policy responses to mitigate its impacts and changes to wages have varied across the world. The likely impacts of inflation on life expectancy trends are also likely to vary as a result. However, the estimates produced earlier for Scotland illustrate that reductions in the real incomes of populations, especially of those already on low incomes, are likely to have large negative impacts on life expectancy, exacerbating the already stagnating and declining trends.

Conclusion

As we have demonstrated earlier in the book, life expectancy trends have stalled across many rich countries, and declined for the poorest groups within countries such as the UK and US. The most important cause of this has been the austerity policies introduced across countries after 2010.[2,64] In this chapter we have introduced three other contributory factors, *two of which apply only from the pandemic onwards.*

Historical rises in obesity across countries are likely to have had a damaging impact on mortality trends, as it is well known that carrying excess weight increases the risks of mortality. However, obesity did not increase in a vacuum. The rise in obesity was due to a wide range of changes in the physical, social and economic environments in which we live, which made it much easier and more likely that we will eat more than we need, and do less physical activity. These changes in turn are due to increased marketisation of our food systems and economy, all of which have promoted unhealthy foods, excessive consumption, technologies that preoccupy us and reduce physical activity, and urban and transport options that revolve around cars. These changes have made our societies more obesogenic: generating and promoting obesity. However, increases in obesity have made only a small contribution to the overall changes in life expectancy trends.

When the pandemic arrived in the UK, it encountered a society with threadbare public services, high rates of poverty and inequality and rising rates of obesity and health conditions. Austerity and the health problems it was creating therefore made us more vulnerable to the impacts of the pandemic, meaning that it killed more people than it would otherwise have done. The measures to control the spread of the virus also had negative health consequences, many of which are only being revealed in the years after 2020. This includes missed medical appointments, interruptions to the education and socialisation of children, social isolation and economic disruption.

As economies opened up, inflation increased quickly, reducing what our money could buy. For populations that have experienced more than ten years of austerity, this has been the last straw for many, causing people to miss out on the essentials needed to keep themselves healthy. Inflation is likely to have pushed life expectancy down further, compounding the impacts of austerity, obesity and the pandemic.

All of these problems – austerity, obesity, the pandemic and inflation – have caused more pain and suffering to those who were already disadvantaged, exacerbating the pre-existing inequalities across society. They are also all still having negative effects now, and can reasonably be expected to have continuing negative impacts for some years to come, even if policies were to change radically and quickly. Unfortunately, austerity responses are once again widely being implemented as we emerge from the pandemic, we still live in obesogenic environments and inflation remains high. Rather than these exposures diminishing, they seem to be ratcheting up.

We are also acutely aware of the health and health-inequality impacts of climate change, and the potential for catastrophic changes in societies as ecological tipping points are breached. Although it does not seem at present that climate change and biodiversity loss are important in explaining the changed life expectancy trends we see at the moment, it seems likely that they will be into the future.[7,60,68,69]

The English Chief Medical Officer, Professor Chris Whitty, gave evidence to the UK COVID Inquiry on 21 November 2023. He said that if there was 'a possibility of 100,000-plus people sadly dying from a terrorist attack', the chances were that a meeting of the UK government's highest-level emergency committee (COBRA) would immediately be convened.

Yet, there are no COBRA meetings for the changed mortality trends. There is no plan to address the problem. There is no independent public inquiry. But many, many, hundreds of thousands of people across the UK have died as a result of the changed mortality trends, many more than died directly from COVID.[70,70,71] The next chapter discusses what the evidence shows would in fact be a commensurate response to this public health emergency.

David

A country's social security system is often described as a 'safety net'. Something we hope not to have to use, but which provides us with the reassurance that it will help us out in times of need – it will catch us if we fall. That wasn't exactly David Clapson's experience of the system.

David could have been described as a very ordinary Englishman. From Stevenage in Hertfordshire, in the Home Counties, as a young man he joined the British army. He rose to Lance Corporal in the Royal Signals, the regiment that provides the army with telecommunications infrastructure. Having thus learned a trade, he left the army after five years, and then spent the next 24 years working for a variety of different companies, including 16 years at British Telecom. However, when his mother was diagnosed with dementia he gave up work to care for her.[1]

After his mother died in 2010, David set about finding a new job with vigour. He signed up for the Job Centre's 'Work Programme' and undertook two unpaid work placements, including one at the retailer B&Q. He also successfully completed a training course to drive a forklift truck. However, he struggled to find suitable full-time employment.

David was described by his sister, Gill Thompson, as a very private and proud person – someone who did not like to rely on charity, or to ask others for help. He desperately wanted to work and had submitted multiple online applications.

However, in May 2013, he missed two appointments with the Job Centre and was consequently 'sanctioned'. As we discussed in Chapter 3, sanctions are punishments given to social security claimants, in which some or all their money is withdrawn for a period of time because they are deemed not to have complied with particular conditions associated with their receipt of benefit – the most common of which is not attending an appointment.[2] While these sanctions pre-date the UK government's austerity programme, major changes to the conditionality of the social security system were introduced in the Welfare Reform Act of 2012.[3-5] In 2022 alone, more than *half a million* sanctions were imposed in the UK, with the average length of sanction being 11–12 weeks (almost three months).[2]

In David's case what this meant that was he would receive no money to live on for a whole month. No money for food, no money to pay bills, no money to live. This is not what anyone could describe as a safety net.

David had Type 1 diabetes. He required daily injections of insulin to survive. Weeks after being sanctioned by the state, and left with nothing to live on, he died. His cause of death was recorded as diabetic ketoacidosis, a complication of diabetes caused by an acute lack of insulin. The fridge where his insulin was stored wasn't working because his electricity had been cut off. His bank account balance was £3.44; his pay-as-you-go mobile phone had 5p credit. His kitchen cupboards contained six tea bags, an out-of-date can of sardines and one tin of soup. The autopsy showed his stomach to be empty.[1]

David's body was found by his sister Gill in his Stevenage flat. A pile of printed-out CVs lay nearby. He was 59 years old.

The Department for Work and Pensions later told Gill: 'we followed procedures; no errors were made'.[6]

As Gill eloquently points out: 'Being vulnerable is not a crime; it is a suffering, and vulnerable people should not be punished, but helped and supported through difficult times'.

The UK social security system didn't catch David when he fell. It caused his fall.

7

What do we need to do?

> We cannot solve a crisis without treating it as a crisis. ... And if solutions within the system are so impossible to find, maybe we should change the system itself.
>
> Greta Thunberg[1]

In this book we have presented the evidence of horrific changes to mortality and life expectancy trends across the UK – changes which have accounted for literally hundreds of thousands of extra deaths. We have shown that while issues such as increases in adult obesity are relevant and important to understand, the principal cause of the changes has been UK government austerity measures.

The title of this book – *Social Murder?* – is deliberately provocative. And we leave it to the reader to decide on an appropriate description of what has occurred in the UK since 2010. However, it is worth repeating part of Friedrich Engels' (who coined the term 'social murder') own definition, which we included in the opening pages of the book:

> when society places hundreds ... in such a position that they inevitably meet a too early and an unnatural death ... when it deprives thousands of the necessaries of life, places them under conditions in which they cannot live ... its deed is murder just as surely as the deed of the single individual.[2]

Engels was describing the appalling living and working conditions – which led directly to appalling *dying* conditions – that were allowed to exist in 19th-century Manchester at the peak of the Industrial Revolution. However, the term 'social murder' has since been applied to a wide variety of settings and events where decisions made by those in power have ultimately caused the deaths of a great many ordinary people. These include the 2017 Grenfell fire in London (as one commentator memorably put it: 'over 170 years after Engels, Britain is still a country that murders its poor'[3]), the actions (or inactions) of governments of many countries in the face of the COVID-19 pandemic, colonialism in South Africa and, of course, the policies put in place in the UK since 2010 – also described by others as 'economic violence'[4] – that we have discussed in depth here.[5–7]

We have discussed how those effects of austerity have been made worse by both the COVID-19 pandemic and subsequent high inflation (the cost-of-living crisis). We have demonstrated that austerity policies have also had detrimental effects on population health in other countries; however, it seems likely that the effects in the UK have been worse than in many other countries because of the particular form austerity has taken here, one which has impacted most on the poorest and most vulnerable among us. We have also discussed the responses to this crisis from those in positions of power and influence, responses which have ranged from (at best) unhelpfulness to (at worst) denial, obfuscation and dereliction of public health duty. In this final chapter we discuss what responses are actually required.

The challenge may seem daunting. The evidence of the changes to mortality rates that we showed in the first two chapters make this clear. Let's look at one last example: this is for females of all ages in Leeds (Figure 7.1). In this chart, the austerity years are shaded grey. Prior to that period, despite some slight fluctuation in rates, mortality levels among women living in the 20 per cent most deprived neighbourhoods of the city had been declining, as we would expect to be the case. However, between 2010/12 and 2018/20, rates *increased* every year. As we discussed in the very first chapter of the book, in a wealthy country like England, this simply should not happen. And the resulting widening gap between those living in the poorest and wealthiest areas is again clear to see. We showed similar widening gaps for all England and all Scotland in Chapter 2, including by means of more sophisticated measures of inequality. The question, therefore, is how do we reverse the widening of these inequalities across the UK?

Narrowing inequalities

The good news is that this is actually a remarkably easy question to answer. It is hard to overstate just how much research has been undertaken into health inequalities – both globally and also just within the UK. Go to any UK public health conference at any point in any year, and look at the programme: it's almost overwhelming. You literally couldn't throw a brick without it hitting either a poster describing research into some form of health inequality, or someone who will be giving a presentation on the subject.[8] This is in part explained by the importance of the topic: it affects all of us, and even governments whose policies have clearly widened inequalities nonetheless talk brazenly of the importance of narrowing them.[9-11] However, it is also explained by the way in which universities appraise the contribution of academics. Researchers have to prove their worth to their employers by obtaining grants to fund research, and then by producing outputs (journal papers, reports, presentations) from that research. Whether this is the optimum model for universities is a discussion for another day; the point

Figure 7.1: Age-standardised mortality rates (ASMRs), females (all ages), Leeds and its 20 per cent most and least deprived neighbourhoods, 1981–2020

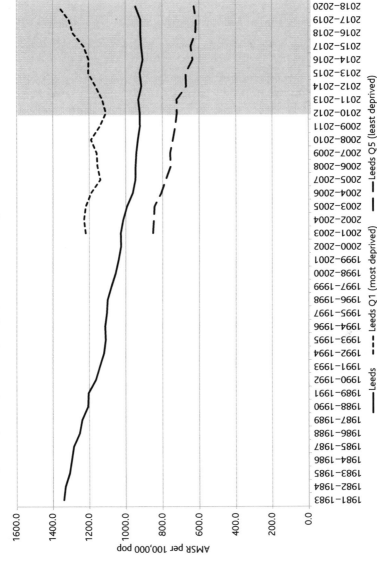

Source: Calculated from ONS mortality and population data

here is that, as a consequence, the evidence base for health inequalities in the UK is enormous. And, importantly, while much of that evidence describes different facets of *the problem* (as our charts in the first two chapters of the book do), there has also been a great deal of research into *the solutions to the problem*.

As with many areas of research, however, the solution–focused evidence base includes a fairly broad spectrum of relevance and usefulness. Over the years – and perhaps again driven by the pressure to continually produce written outputs in one form or another – there has been a fair bit of hand-wringing in academic journals with regard to the complexity of health inequalities. A number of papers have described them as a 'wicked issue' – not in the sense of them being immoral (which they clearly are) but in the sense that they are seen as a problem that is so hard to solve.[12-15] This has been echoed by entirely unevidenced proclamations by some of the same think-tanks discussed in Chapter 5. For example, in a high-profile report on health inequalities in Scotland published in 2023, the Health Foundation chose to ignore important evidence for effective solutions and instead declared that it was not just the responsibility of governments to address such inequalities but that it was, rather, down to all of us: 'This is a problem for every one of us … each of us has our part to play'[16] This is nonsense. All the evidence shows that health inequalities are entirely political in nature and they therefore require entirely political solutions.[17-24] To the extent that this is 'down to us' (in the words of the Health Foundation), it is only in respect to whether or not we wield our collective power as a population (for example, through voting, political party membership, protests and campaigns, participation in trade unions, the use of our spending power and so on) to ensure that people who make decisions do so to benefit us all.

Returning to the academic research, while it may indeed be a complex or a 'wicked' problem to understand, for example, whether a particular small-scale initiative in a particular neighbourhood will impact on a particular aspect of inequality (for example, what will be the impact on well-being of the creation of a community garden in a run-down area?), at the level of whole populations – across all society – we actually already know well what interventions are effective in narrowing health inequalities and which are not. We know what works.[25-28]

Several years ago NHS Health Scotland (which has since morphed into Public Health Scotland) published a review of all the international evidence of what works to narrow health inequalities.[26] It demonstrated that policies are required at three levels: socioeconomic inequalities; the physical and social environment; and individual experiences.

First and foremost, because of the link between socioeconomic inequalities and health inequalities that we discussed in Chapter 3, you need policies which make society more equal in the first place: do that, and health inequalities will narrow as a consequence. So, you need policies which address why there are such wide socioeconomic inequalities in society. This means reducing the concentration of wealth and power (and the resulting flows of rent, profit, interest and so on – all of which move income from poorer to richer groups[29,30]), eliminating poverty, introducing progressive taxation (that is, the 'Robin Hood' method of taking more from the rich and giving more to the poor), providing a comprehensive, generous and unconditional social security system and introducing labour market legislation to help the low-paid.

At the second level, policies in relation to broader 'environmental' factors such as housing, education, health and social care services, clean air and water, neighbourhood quality and transport are important.

Finally, 'third level' policies should target particular individuals' experiences of inequality: for example, measures to help those at particular risk, such as the homeless and children in care.

But the most important part of the evidence presented in the report was this. If you don't address the first level – if you don't make society more equal to start with – you simply won't narrow health inequalities: '*action to address [the other levels] is important, but will not solve the problem*'.[26]

The example of recent policy making in Scotland is quite telling in this regard. While many would argue that the Scottish Government could, and should, have done a lot more with the powers at their disposal in recent times, in fact they have introduced a good number of helpful, and relevant, policies, ones which contrast markedly with the actions of the UK government. However, these have been principally at those second and third levels, rather than the first. Policies such as the expansion of social house-building, more free childcare, free bus travel for children and young adults, minimum pricing of alcohol, and more, have all been introduced.[31] However, like the devolved administrations in Wales and Northern Ireland, the Scottish Government lacks the legislative ability to meaningfully address the first, and most important, level: for the key economic policy areas such as government borrowing, employment legislation, most taxation and the vast majority of social security benefits are all 'reserved' to Westminster. On their own, therefore, the Scottish Government's policies since 2010 would have been unlikely to have meaningfully narrowed health inequalities; but in any case, any benefits have been completely overshadowed by the UK government's policies of austerity – policies (such as the astonishing scale of cuts to social security) which operate at that first level.

Narrowing inequalities – and undoing austerity

That NHS Health Scotland report was published in 2013, just before the evidence of the changing trends in life expectancy emerged.[26] And such has been the scale of those changes, and their impact in terms of massively widening health inequalities, that the need for action is greater than ever: arguably we need to go beyond what was outlined in 2013. Again, however, we don't lack the knowledge of what is required. A coalition of voices has been calling for meaningful change for some time now. In our evidence review published in 2022,[32] no fewer than 40 different policy recommendations were set out, based on proposals from the likes of Oxfam, the Joseph Rowntree Foundation (JRF), the Child Poverty Action Group and more. For the sake of brevity, we do not go through all 40 in any detail here.

At their core, however, were important 'first level' actions: creating a more equal society in the UK and, as part of that, protecting the poorest and most vulnerable. As such, they were about *reversing the policy measures introduced since 2010* – but also going further than that, as health inequalities in 2010 were already wide (for example, wider in Scotland than in any other Western European nation)[33,34] and have since, obviously, widened further.[35]

So they also include the need to *reverse the current concentration of wealth and power* in the hands of a tiny minority, whether that be in relation to ownership of newspapers, internet shopping and social media sites, or houses for private rent.[29,30,36,37] This concentration of wealth and power has been at the root of widening socioeconomic inequalities since the late 1970s/early 1980s, as it creates a flow of money from poorer to richer groups from profits and rents.[30,38-40] The alternative is *economic democracy*, where wealth is owned by us all (after all, we have collectively created the wealth) and is used for the public good.[36,37,41,42] As a step towards democratising wealth ownership, policies which stop tax evasion and avoidance, and increase taxation of wealth, assets (for example, property, investments) and corporate profits can all help. Put simply, if we want to reduce socioeconomic inequalities, then (as sociologist Andrew Sayer's book stated), '*we can't afford the rich*', because it is their wealth and power that generates these flows of income from poor to rich (for example, through rental income on property they own).[30]

The additional revenue from such actions can be used to help create a *social security system* which does what a social security system is supposed to do: be a robust safety net for people in times of need; help people who need help; protect people who need protection. As the Child Poverty Action Group made clear,[43] such a system needs to ensure that people do not fall into poverty, particularly those with additional costs in terms of childcare or having a disability. It needs to protect the income (and therefore the health) of everyone when adverse circumstances occur – such as unemployment, relationship breakdown or becoming ill. It should also be promoted as a service (or safety net) for us *all* – not perceived or portrayed in a stigmatising fashion as something that exists only for certain sections of the population. Despite the screaming tabloid headlines that frequently suggest otherwise, social security levels in the UK are among the lowest in Western Europe.[44,45]

That needs to be changed. Levels of social security benefits need to be increased markedly; the horrors of conditionality (that so affected David Clapson and many like him) need to be reduced or removed. The system itself needs to incorporate values such as dignity and respect, but also efficiency – everything that Moira Dury never experienced.

We also need changes to improve people's *working lives*. There is a solid evidence base that *good* work is positive for health. This means sufficient pay, work availability, job security and quality of employment.[46,47] In terms of wages, currently over 70 per cent of children living in poverty in the UK live in a house where at least one adult works:[48] that tells you a lot about the inadequate levels of wages for so many people. Therefore we need to both increase wages – increasing the statutory minimum wage (the so-called 'living wage', which isn't really a living wage[49]) to the level of the *Real* Living Wage (as set annually by the Living Wage Foundation[50]) is an obvious first step – and increase the value of in-work social security payments (such as the [correctly] much maligned Universal Credit benefit) to prevent families falling into poverty. We also need to support those families' ability to earn adequate wages by providing enough high-quality, funded, childcare places for their children. Employees also need to be safe at work: minimising health and safety risks is vital, as is protection by unions. Unions have been shown to reduce work-related injuries and poor health;[51] restrictions on unions therefore act as an impediment to achieving such reductions. We should promote unions in those terms, not vilify them in the media for seeking to protect workers' rights and well-being. More broadly, in a civilised society, work should offer security, fulfilment and respect: this is the vision of the Fair Work Framework, which should be a blueprint for any government.[52]

We also need to go further in addressing the unacceptable levels of poverty that exist in UK society today. In a country as wealthy as the UK, food banks should simply not exist. There should be no need for them. They have become normalised when they should be abnormal. In the early days of austerity in the UK, Danny Alexander, the then Liberal Democrat Chief Secretary to the Treasury in the Coalition government, was pictured in the media proudly posing at his local food bank, as if carrying out some perverse political version of 'show and tell' ('look what I've made!').[53] Many other politicians have since followed suit. But our political leaders should be standing up to announce the end of food banks, not their continued existence or expansion. To reach that goal, we need to eliminate so-called '*food insecurity*'. This was defined in Chapter 3, and basically means hunger. And hunger is surely completely unacceptable in one of the richest countries in the world.[54] As food banks hardly existed prior to austerity being implemented,[55] it cannot be beyond even the half-brightest political brain to figure out a way to return to pre-2010 levels. We also need to eradicate *fuel poverty*: defined as having to spend a high percentage of your income on household energy (including, in particular, on keeping warm), this again simply should not exist in a modern UK. Increased wages and social security, alongside strategies to address cold and damp housing with affordable heating, better ventilation and energy–efficiency measures, would go a long way to achieving this aim.[56,57] The expansion of housing quality standards (measures used to assess the quality of socially rented housing) would also be important, especially in the private rented sector. More broadly (and especially in England) there is a desperate need for more affordable social housing; the JRF's call for a 'living rent'[58] to match a real living wage could make a big difference to that.

The evidence of the devastating impact of cuts to *public services* has been laid out in different parts of this book, including in some of the individual stories such as those of Paul and Rachel. Properly funded public services (including different social services) are vital for preventing poor health and early death. However, the key words in that last sentence are 'properly' and 'funded'. We need to ensure that everyone in society has access to the services they need, but that there is an additional focus on (and therefore investment in) the areas of greatest need: the areas with more poverty and associated challenges, which are also the areas (as explained in Chapter 3) that have been the worst affected by austerity. This is the concept of so–called 'proportionate universalism': services for all, but greater provision where they are most needed.[27]

It goes without saying that all this goes hand in hand with the need for governmental *macroeconomic policy* which avoids austerity. It's desperately important that politicians understand, and do not ignore, the evidence of the damage that austerity inflicts.

Finally, we have discussed the (lesser) contribution of *obesity* to the overall stalling of improvement in mortality rates and life expectancy. Again, there's an important point to be made here: we have lots of evidence of what influences obesity levels in society, and we know what actions would be successful in reducing them. In 2007 a UK government report mapped out all the many factors that determine obesity.[59] The report is well known in public health circles for a rather bewildering diagram (or 'obesity system map') the authors created: that's not a criticism; the diagram deliberately captures the complexity of it all. As discussed in the previous chapter, obesity is determined not just by how much people eat and/or exercise: lots of factors conspire to create that so-called obesogenic environment. Food production and promotion, the cost of healthy and unhealthy food, poverty levels, how we have been brought up, the environment we live in, the type of job we do, the influence of the media, and lots, lots more are all important. And they are the same areas where good policy making would make a difference: restricting advertising of, and taxing, unhealthy goods, creating an environment which encourages physical activity, making healthy food more affordable and available. It's not rocket science, even if the report's main diagram does bear more than a passing resemblance to a complex planetary system in a galaxy far, far away.

The cost of change

Speaking of other planets, the uncosted nature of all these recommendations will no doubt prompt accusations that we are living on one. In these post-pandemic days of high inflation, how could the country possibly afford to create the kind of society we have outlined? Again, the answer is not a difficult one. First, many of the proposals outlined here (for example, taxation measures) would actually *raise* income for the government. Second, as we have stated on multiple occasions, the UK is a very, very wealthy society. It's just that the wealth is extraordinarily unequally distributed. For example, in 2023, the 50 richest families in the UK had more wealth than half of the UK population combined (that's more than the wealth of 33 million people).[60] Multiple measures could be implemented to make society more equal and which could better protect the health of the majority, not just continue to protect the wealth of the few. Given the political history of the UK, it would of course require a dramatic change in government policy.

However, it's worth reflecting on what prompted a very recent, equally dramatic, change in UK government policy. The COVID-19 pandemic elicited an extraordinary response from the UK Conservative government (and, of course, from other governments around the world). As was alluded to in the previous chapter, billions were spent on protecting people's incomes through the furlough scheme, and credit is also due for the increase ('uplift') in the value of key social security benefits, including Universal Credit (albeit that, shamefully, the increase was later reversed – in the face of good evidence of the poverty increase and associated poor health that would result[61–64]). And, of course, the billions spent include an estimated £10 billion that was wasted on contracts for unusable, non-existent or over-priced healthcare equipment, including those allegedly given to friends of government ministers.[65,66] Nonetheless, an extraordinary amount of money was spent on seeking to protect the health of the population – and, in doing so, ensuring that the National Health Service could cope with what would otherwise have been unmanageable demands (even more so than did happen). This was all prompted by statistical modelling analyses published in March 2020 which suggested that, without taking preventative action (instigating social and economic lockdowns and so on), around half a million people would die from COVID-19,[67] reducing life expectancy in the UK by almost six years.

However, inequality in the UK already accounts for a loss of 3.5 years of life expectancy *each year*. In other words, *every couple of years* inequality in the UK results in a loss of life greater than the scale of an unmitigated

COVID-19 pandemic – the scale of which so spooked the UK government into this unprecedented policy response.[68] Furthermore, as we discussed in Chapters 1 and 3, more people have died from austerity than from COVID-19. So, if a dramatic political response to save lives was possible in response to a pandemic, why can a different – but similarly dramatic and unprecedented – response not be possible in relation to factors that cause even more deaths in UK society?

What now?

Returning to the policy recommendations, there are clearly many more, very specific, measures that we could list and discuss here – but they have been outlined in detail elsewhere[32] and do not need to be repeated. And we have also not delved deeply into the important differences between what can be done at UK government level and the much more limited capabilities of the devolved Scottish, Welsh and Northern Irish governments. But, to repeat the most important point: we know what to do; the question is whether those with the autonomy to act will do so. And returning to the first level of required policy actions, it's political will at UK government level that matters the most. That is where the vast majority of economic powers currently lie.

To change our politics as already described (to help influence and bring about this political will), we need to use the power we have when we act collectively. This does mean voting carefully (and remembering to take your identification with you to the polling station on polling day), but it means much more too. To really change our politics we need to be active citizens: building campaigns and protests; creating and supporting institutions and organisations that can help (whether they be specific campaign groups, alternative media, trades unions, tenants' groups, disability rights groups, workers' co-operatives and so on); if we have money to spend, spending it wisely so that it helps rather than hinders economic inequalities; and more.

At the time of writing, a UK general election is a matter of months away. The polls predict an end to the government which has inflicted austerity on UK society and instead foresee a Labour administration under the leadership of Sir Keir Starmer. Would that mean an end to austerity? Better, would it mean a *reversal* of austerity? Better still, would it mean the introduction of the types of policies laid out in this chapter which would protect the poorest, promote equality and ultimately save lives?

The signs don't look particularly good. Even the biggest champion of the Labour Party would have to admit that their approach thus far has been cautious in the extreme. A great many of the policies that formed the backbone of Starmer's personal election campaign (to become leader of the party in 2020) have been – or seem likely to be – abandoned: increasing income tax for the top 5 per cent of earners, abolishing Universal Credit, returning key services (rail, mail, energy and water) to public ownership, scrapping charitable status for private schools, and more. More worryingly, the Party has publicly stated that they will not reverse the social security two-child benefits cap that was discussed in Chapter 3 – a policy seen in many ways as emblematic of austerity, and described by one eminent academic and commentator as 'the worst social security policy ever'.[69] Loyal Party members have expressed emotions ranging from serious concern to downright consternation at this pronouncement.[70,71]

However, while Keir Starmer may have his critics (and their number may well have increased on the back of such recent announcements), Anne-Marie O'Sullivan is not one of them. Anne-Marie is the daughter of Michael O'Sullivan – the man whose story began this book. Anne-Marie has spent the years since her father's tragic death seeking some form of justice: trying to have an inquiry established by the Parliamentary and Health Service Ombudsman into the actions of the Department for Work and Pensions (DWP) of the UK government which ultimately led to her Dad taking his own life. In effect, she has been trying to have the DWP admit their guilt. As one might imagine, such an attempt to fight the system is not an easy one. However, she has had a strong ally in the form of her local MP: Keir Starmer. And Anne-Marie speaks movingly of all the help she has received from him. She talks warmly of his 'compassion' and 'decency', of his understanding of the details of her father's case and, therefore, of the impact that the policies of austerity have had on individuals like Michael. However, what we need now is for political leaders like Keir Starmer to understand not just the politically caused *individual* tragedies of Michael and others featured in this book – Rachel, Frances, Paul, Moira, Ellen and David – but also to understand what these policies have done *collectively* to the society in which we all live: a society where wealth abounds, but where child poverty is rampant, food banks proliferate and extraordinary numbers of our fellow citizens die before their time. We need them to examine and understand the evidence of how this has happened, and to use that evidence as a basis for not just reversing the policies of austerity but fundamentally making society a better and more caring place.

If poverty in a wealthy country is a political choice, as Philip Alston so eloquently pointed out, then so too is *no poverty*. It is not only within the gift of our political leaders to achieve this: it is surely their moral obligation.

APPENDIX

Summary of the causal evidence that austerity has led to the mortality trend changes

Table A1 summarises the published studies that have demonstrated a causal relationship between austerity and mortality. We have limited this list to quantitative studies in which all-cause mortality or life expectancy was the outcome, and where the study design included at least two comparison groups (that is, more versus less exposed to austerity). We have therefore not included the numerous studies of the impacts of austerity on mental health or on specific causes of death such as suicide.

The extent to which any research demonstrates that one thing causes another has been the subject of many medical, public health and economic texts.[1-7] The Bradford-Hill considerations are often regarded as the starting point for deciding whether something is a cause – and these have been elaborated upon by many other authors since.[8] Key to demonstrating causality is:

1. There must be a (statistical) relationship between the cause and effect (in this instance, austerity and mortality) which is not due to some other interfering factor (most commonly called 'confounding' in this form of research).
2. The cause must come before the effect.
3. Changes in the cause must give rise to changes in the outcome (that is, if austerity is introduced, does this impact on mortality trends?).

The most convincing way to demonstrate causality is to undertake an experiment in which the researcher introduces the suggested cause to a random selection of subjects. This would be the form of evidence generated in experiments of the effectiveness of medicines.

For austerity, this is impossible because researchers do not have control over whether such policies are implemented or not in society. Instead, evaluation methods are used to ensure that the observed effects (of different political and economic decisions being made across countries and over time) are not due to other factors.[7] This becomes an even more convincing evidence base when different research groups, studying different populations, and using different data and different methods (which generate different potential forms of bias) all find similar results.[5,6] And this is precisely what Table A1 shows.

Table A1: Summary of the evidence that austerity has caused the change in mortality trends

Study	Population	Study design	Austerity measure	Outcome	Biases accounted for	Findings
Alexiou 2021[9]	English local authorities (2013–17)	Panel regression study	Local government funding	Life expectancy and mortality	• Biases between areas that don't change over time • Most likely sources of bias that change over time	Every £100 per person cut in local government funding led to 1.3 months' decline in life expectancy, with the average funding cut being £168 over the 4 years, equating to a decline of 2.2 months of life expectancy.
Beckfield 2016[10]	High-income countries (1971–2010)	Panel regression study	Welfare benefit generosity	Life expectancy	• Biases between areas that don't change over time • Most likely sources of bias that change over time	Increases in welfare generosity led to increases in life expectancy.
Loopstra 2017[11]	English local authorities (2007–13)	Ecological study of changes over time	Pension Credit and social care spending changes	Mortality	• Biases between areas that don't change over time	Each 1% cut in Pension Credit spending led to a 0.68% increase in mortality.
Martin 2021[12]	English local authorities (2010/11–2014/15)	Regression using instrumental variables	Healthcare, social care and local public health spending	Mortality	• Biases between areas that don't change over time • Most likely sources of bias that change over time	Changes to spending on healthcare, social care and public health led to over 57,000 extra deaths between 2010/11 and 2014/15 in England (immediate impacts only counted).
McCartney 2022[13]	High-income countries (2000–19)	Panel regression study	Cyclically-Adjusted Primary Balance (CAPB), Alesina-Ardagna Fiscal Index (AAFI), public social spending, and government expenditure as % of GDP	Life expectancy, mortality, age-specific mortality, lifespan variation	• Biases between areas that don't change over time • Most likely sources of bias that change over time	Austerity worsened mortality across 3 of 4 measures, with large negative impacts across all measures when austerity was implemented during economic downturns.

(continued)

Table A1: Summary of the evidence that austerity has caused the change in mortality trends (continued)

Study	Population	Study design	Austerity measure	Outcome	Biases accounted for	Findings
Prędkiewicz 2022[14]	European countries (1995–2019)	Panel regression study	Government budget balance	Life expectancy	• Biases between areas that don't change over time • Biases over time were checked with an alternative model	Austerity is harmful for male and female life expectancy.
Rajmil 2019[15]	European countries (2011–15)	Panel regression study	Cyclically-Adjusted Primary Balance (CAPB)	Excess mortality	• Biases between areas that don't change over time	Compared to the lowest austerity third of countries, the intermediate and high austerity countries had excess mortality rates of 40 and 31 deaths per 100,000 population, respectively, in 2015.
Seaman 2023[16]	Great Britain (2011–16)	Panel regression study	Change in social security spending	Life expectancy	• Biases between areas that don't change over time • Most likely sources of bias that change over time	For every £100 of cut per head in social security, there was a loss of 1 month of life expectancy.[17]
Toffolutti 2019[18]	European countries (1991–2013)	Panel regression study	Alesina-Ardagna Fiscal Index	Mortality	• Biases between areas that don't change over time	Austerity led to a 0.7% increase in mortality.
Watkins 2017[19]	English local authorities (2011–14)	Panel regression study	Healthcare and social care spending changes	Mortality	• Biases between areas that don't change over time	Cuts to health and social care spending in England led to 45,000 extra deaths between 2011 and 2014.

The table provides details of the study design and which forms of 'interference' (or confounding) each study was able to take into account. Most of the studies here are 'panel regression studies', which means that they use data from a large number of areas (for example, countries or local authorities), over a number of years, and check whether changes in austerity between areas, or within areas, can explain changes in the outcomes. Usually these studies also ensure that the cause (austerity) comes before the effect (mortality or life expectancy).

Overall, these studies provide clear evidence that austerity has caused the changes in mortality trends.

Notes and references

Epigraph

1 Engels F. The Condition of the Working Class in England. Oxford: Oxford University Press, 2009.

2 Chakrabortty A. Over 170 years after Engels, Britain is still a country that murders its poor. *The Guardian.* 2017; published online 20 June. https://www.theguardian.com/commentisfree/2017/jun/20/engels-britain-murders-poor-grenfell-tower.

3 Blakely G. Capitalism has always been authoritarian. *Tribune.* 2023; published online March. https://tribunemag.co.uk/2021/03/capitalism-has-always-been-authoritarian.

Chapter 1

1 O'Sullivan A-M. Personal communication. 2023.

2 McVeigh K. 'Fitness to work' assessments are brutal, says daughter of man who killed himself. *The Guardian.* 2015; published online 22 Oct. https://www.theguardian.com/society/2015/oct/22/fitness-to-work-assessments-are-brutal-says-daughter-of-man-who-killed-himself.

3 Pring J. Michael O'Sullivan scandal: DWP twice pushed dad-of-two to suicide bids. *Disability News Service.* 2015; published online 23 Oct. https://www.disabilitynewsservice.com/michael-osullivan-scandal-dwp-twice-pushed-dad-of-two-to-suicide-bids/.

4 Kennedy S. Incapacity benefit reassessments. London: House of Commons Library, 2014 https://researchbriefings.files.parliament.uk/documents/SN06855/SN06855.pdf.

5 These assessments ('work capability assessments' [WCAs]) were introduced by the previous Labour UK Government in 2008. However, the Conservative-Liberal Democrat coalition introduced a process of 'reassessment' in 2010, initially affecting around 1.5 million people in the UK.

6 Scottish Government. Welfare Reform (Further Provision) (Scotland) Act 2012: annual report 2017. Edinburgh: Scottish Government, 2017.

7 Gillon D. How Atos comes under pressure to declare disabled people as fit for work. *The Guardian.* 2013; published online Dec 9. https://www.theguardian.com/commentisfree/2013/dec/09/atos-disabled-people-assessment-fit-work-report.

8 Gentleman A. Why I blew the whistle on Atos fitness-for-work test. *The Guardian.* 2013; published online 31 July. https://www.theguardian.com/society/2013/jul/31/atos-fitness-work-test-greg-wood.

9   Bloom D. Disability benefit assessors trouser £50 rewards for squeezing extra tests into their day. *The Mirror*. 2018; published online 14 March. https://www.mirror.co.uk/news/politics/disability-benefit-assessors-trouser-50-12535091.

10 The calculation of ASMRs takes into account both the age of those dying and the age of the population where they lived: obviously an area with an older population will usually experience more deaths than an area with a younger population, and ASMRs are just a way of taking this into account so the rates can be meaningfully compared.

11 Statisticians and epidemiologists will be bristling at this over-simplification – but it's effectively true. The 'official' definition of life expectancy (or 'period life expectancy at birth', to give it its proper name) is 'the average number of years a new-born is expected to live if current mortality rates continue to apply'. However – and this is the whole point of this book – mortality rates shouldn't (and usually don't) stay the same, they change over time. So this definition is really quite unhelpful, and thinking of life expectancy as a rough indication of the ages that people are currently dying at (or living to) makes a lot more sense.

12 Max Planck Institute for Demographic Research, University of California, Berkeley, French Institute for Demographic Studies. Human Mortality Database. www.mortality.org (accessed 9 Aug 2023).

13 Figure 1.1 shows changes in overall life expectancy (for males and females combined) in England and Wales (dark line) and Scotland (lighter line) between 1900/02 (when life expectancy in England and Wales was only around 48 years) and 2017/19 (when it was about 81 years in England and Wales).

14 When the health of a population improves, ASMRs come down (because there are fewer deaths per year) and life expectancy goes up (because people are living longer as a result).

15 The 'Spanish' Influenza pandemic of 1918–19, and the more recent COVID-19 pandemic.

16 Walsh D, McCartney G, Minton J, Parkinson J, Shipton D, Whyte B. Changing mortality trends in countries and cities of the UK: a population-based trend analysis. *BMJ Open* 2020; **10**: e038135.

17 Figure 1.2 shows the trend in life expectancy between 1980/82 and 2017/19 for females (dark line) and males (lighter line) in Scotland (top chart) and England and Wales (bottom chart). The change in trends from the early 2010s is evident in all four lines shown.

18 Walsh D, McCartney G. *Changing mortality rates in Scotland and the UK: an updated summary*. Glasgow: Glasgow Centre for Population Health, 2023 https://www.gcph.co.uk/assets/0000/9348/Changing_mortality_rates_in_Scotland_and_the_UK_-_an_updated_summary_FINAL.pdf.

19 Figure 1.3 shows the trend in ASMRs for females living in Scotland (top chart) and England (bottom chart), respectively, between 1981/83 and 2017/19. In both cases, the solid line represents the rates for all females living in their respective countries, while the short-dashed line shows the rates for those living in neighbourhoods classed as the 20 per cent most socioeconomically deprived, and the long-dashed line the rates for those living in the 20 per cent least deprived areas. For reasons of data availability, the trends for the most and least deprived areas cover the period from 2001 onwards only. The change in rates in, especially, the most deprived areas from the early 2010s is very evident.

20 Figure 1.4 shows similar mortality rates (ASMRs) to those shown in Figure 1.3, but this time just for the city of Glasgow (and its 20 per cent most and least deprived neighbourhoods), and only for females aged under 65 years.

21 Walsh D, Dundas R, McCartney G, Gibson M, Seaman R. Bearing the burden of austerity: how do changing mortality rates in the UK compare between men and women? *Journal of Epidemiology and Community Health* 2022; **76**: 1027.

Rachel

1 Lambert G. Thousands of people admitted to hospital with malnutrition. *The Times*. 2023; published online 10 July. https://www.thetimes.co.uk/article/times-health-commission-thousands-of-people-admitted-to-hospital-suffering-from-malnutrition-n23hqgzjr.

2 *Deaths due to malnutrition*. London: Office for National Statistics, 2022 https://www.ons.gov.uk/aboutus/transparencyandgovernance/freedomofinformationfoi/deathsduetomalnutrition.

3 Ryan F. *Crippled: austerity and the demonization of disabled people*. London: Verso, 2019.

4 Rachel's story is adapted from Frances Ryan's book (*Crippled: austerity and the demonization of disabled people*) with permission and grateful thanks.

5 Osborne G. George Osborne's speech to the Conservative party conference in full. *The Guardian*. 2010; published online 4 Oct. https://www.theguardian.com/politics/2010/oct/04/george-osborne-speech-conservative-conference.

6 Gray M, Barford A. The depths of the cuts: the uneven geography of local government austerity. *Cambridge Journal of Regions, Economy and Society* 2018; **11**: 541–63.

7 Taylor-Robinson D, Gosling R. Local authority budget cuts and health inequalities. *BMJ* 2011; **342**: d1487.

8 Alexiou A, Fahy K, Mason K, et al. Local government funding and life expectancy in England: a longitudinal ecological study. *The Lancet Public Health* 2021; **6**: e641–7.

Chapter 2

1 McCartney G, Walsh D, Whyte B, Collins C. Has Scotland always been the 'sick man' of Europe? An observational study from 1855 to 2006. *European Journal of Public Health* 2012; **22**: 756–60.

2 Mackenbach JP. Convergence and divergence of life expectancy in Europe: a centennial view. *European Journal of Epidemiology* 2013; **28**: 229–40.

3 Not least because – as we will go on to explain – the biggest changes have been seen among poorer populations where life expectancy is nowhere near any such 'natural limit'. In the poorest 20 per cent neighbourhoods of Glasgow, for example (data for which were shown in Figure 1.4 in the previous chapter), male life expectancy prior to the pandemic was 73.6 years: that's the figure that was recorded for the UK in 1980, almost 45 years ago (see reference 1).And while Glasgow has often been the subject of the most striking headlines regarding low life expectancy in the UK, similarly, almost-but-not-quite-so-appalling, figures can be shown for the poorer parts of just about any UK town or city.

4 Walsh D, Tod E, McCartney G, Levin KA. How much of the stalled mortality trends in Scotland and England can be attributed to obesity? *BMJ Open* 2022; **12**: e067310.

5 We use this age group because this was one of the age bands used in the study. However, a very similar trend can be seen for all ages, not just 15–84 years.

6 Sparing the reader unwanted statistical jargon, the linear trend here is effectively the slope of the line that is represented by the data points. Statisticians would provide a much better, more complex definition, but you wouldn't necessarily thank them for it.

7 Note that the chart shows rates for each individual year, rather than for the three-year averages used in the figures in Chapter 1. Because death rates normally fluctuate slightly year by year, for the charts in Chapter 1 (and elsewhere in the book) we smoothed the lines by showing three-year average figures (for example, the average life expectancy for 1981–83, rather than the values for the individual years 1981, 1982, 1983). That can help the clarity of charts, which is especially important for interpreting long-term trends. Nonetheless, some people worry that this approach can mask potentially important year-specific variation. We take a pragmatic approach of showing both versions of the trends, depending on the context and the source material from which the data have been taken. In the example here, having year-by-year data is important because the linear trend has been fitted to those individual, year-specific, data points.

8 Minton J, Fletcher E, Ramsay J, Little K, McCartney G. How bad are life expectancy trends across the UK, and what would it take to get back to previous trends? *Journal of Epidemiology and Community Health* 2020; **74**: 741.

9   Similar to Figure 2.1, Figure 2.2 again compares values predicted by previous trends with what actually happened. Here, the figure shows life expectancy rather than mortality rates, and shows the data for only the most recent period in question (2012–18). Each pair of panels are for the four UK nations, with the panels on the left for females and those on the right for males. The black, solid, line represents the level of life expectancy in the period 2012–18 that is predicted by previous trends in the years 1990–2011, while the squares are the actual life expectancy values in each year. The grey, dotted lines (technically the 5th and 95th percentiles) in effect signify a likely range of accuracy for the predictions.

10   Walsh D, Dundas R, McCartney G, Gibson M, Seaman R. Bearing the burden of austerity: how do changing mortality rates in the UK compare between men and women? *Journal of Epidemiology and Community Health* 2022; **76**: 1027.

11   Darlington-Pollock F, Green MA, Simpson L. Why were there 231,707 more deaths than expected in England between 2010 and 2018? An ecological analysis of mortality records. *Journal of Public Health* 2022; **44**: 310–18.

12   Darlington-Pollok et al's estimate of c. 232,000 excess deaths for England only, in 2010–18, is very similar our own estimate of c. 250,000 deaths for England and Wales for 2012–18. Other estimates (such as by Martin et al) are included in the next chapter.

13   Fenton L, Minton J, Ramsay J, et al. Recent adverse mortality trends in Scotland: comparison with other high-income countries. *BMJ Open* 2019; **9**: e029936.

14   McCartney G, McMaster R, Popham F, Dundas R, Walsh D. Is austerity a cause of slower improvements in mortality in high-income countries? A panel analysis. *Social Science & Medicine* 2022; **313**: 115397.

15   This may exceed the bounds of readers' interest, but the statistical technique is called segmented regression. It's a fairly sophisticated way of identifying so-called 'break points' in time trend data (that is, the points at which the trend changed) based on changes to the slope of the line. Importantly, it can assess whether the changes are meaningful ('significant' in COD-statistical language) or instead more likely to be just the result of chance.

16   As with Figure 2.1, in Figure 2.3 the dots represent the actual mortality rates in each year, and the solid lines are the regression lines that have been 'fitted' to the data. Unlike in Figure 2.1, however, here two regression lines have been drawn for every series of data, one before and one after the change in trend (in the published study, segmented regression [explained in note 15] was again used to identify these breaks in the trends). On each chart 'Q1' represents the most deprived quintile (that is, 20 per cent) of the population and Q5 the least deprived quintile.

17 Walsh D, McCartney G. *Changing mortality rates in Scotland and the UK: an updated summary.* Glasgow: Glasgow Centre for Population Health, 2023 https://www.gcph.co.uk/assets/0000/9348/Changing_mortality_rates_in_Scotland_and_the_UK_-_an_updated_summary_FINAL.pdf.

18 Figure 2.3 shows ASMRs between 1981 and 2019 for Scotland (top two charts) and England (bottom two charts), shown separately for males (on the left) and females (on the right). As with previous figures, rates are shown for everyone from 1981, and for those living in the 20 per cent most and least socioeconomically deprived areas of each country from 2001. As was the case in Figure 2.1, linear trend lines have been fitted to (drawn through) the data points (mortality rates).

19 Figure 2.4 presents similar data to those shown for Glasgow in Figure 1.4 in Chapter 1 (mortality rates for those aged under 65 years) between 1981/ 83 and 2017/19, but this time for males in four English cities (Leeds, Liverpool, Bristol and Sheffield), including trends for each city's 20 per cent most and least socioeconomically deprived neighbourhoods (shown for 2001 onwards). As in Glasgow, changes in (previously decreasing) mortality trends in the most deprived areas are very evident from the early 2010s.

20 Walsh D, McCartney G, Minton J, Parkinson J, Shipton D, Whyte B. Changing mortality trends in countries and cities of the UK: a population-based trend analysis. *BMJ Open* 2020; **10**: e038135.

21 Currie J, Schilling HT, Evans L, et al. Contribution of avoidable mortality to life expectancy inequalities in Wales: a decomposition by age and by cause between 2002 and 2020. *Journal of Public Health* 2022; published online Nov. DOI:10.1093/pubmed/fdac133.

22 Fenton L, Wyper GM, McCartney G, Minton J. Socioeconomic inequality in recent adverse all-cause mortality trends in Scotland. *Journal of Epidemiology and Community Health* 2019; **73**: 971.

23 Rashid T, Bennett JE, Paciorek CJ, et al. Life expectancy and risk of death in 6791 communities in England from 2002 to 2019: high-resolution spatiotemporal analysis of civil registration data. *The Lancet Public Health* 2021; **6**: e805–16.

24 Bennett JE, Pearson-Stuttard J, Kontis V, Capewell S, Wolfe I, Ezzati M. Contributions of diseases and injuries to widening life expectancy inequalities in England from 2001 to 2016: a population-based analysis of vital registration data. *The Lancet Public Health* 2018; **3**: e586–97.

25 These are based on the respective indices of 'multiple deprivation' used in each country, which classify and rank small neighbourhoods in terms of a broad set of socioeconomic indicators related to, for example, income, employment, education, crime and housing. Although the Scottish and English indices are separate, and use different indicators and differently sized neighbourhoods, they are very similar in terms of their basic composition, and thus broadly comparable.

26 Shorrocks A, Davies J, Lluberas R. Global Wealth Report 2022. Zürich: Credit Suisse, 2022 https://www.credit-suisse.com/about-us/en/reports-research/global-wealth-report.html.

27 OECD. *Income inequality*. https://data.oecd.org/inequality/income-ine quality.htm.

28 Dransfield S. *A tale of two Britains: inequality in the UK*. Oxford: Oxfam UK, 2014.

29 Ramsay J, Minton J, Fischbacher C, et al. How have changes in death by cause and age group contributed to the recent stalling of life expectancy gains in Scotland? Comparative decomposition analysis of mortality data, 2000–2002 to 2015–2017. *BMJ Open* 2020; **10**: e036529.

30 *A review of recent trends in mortality in England*. London: Public Health England, 2018.

31 Figure 2.5 compares the change in life expectancy in the period 2000/02 to 2012/14 (dark bars) with the change between 2012/14 and 2015/17 (light bars) – by age group. In the first time period, life expectancy in each age group increased (especially among some of the older age bands) – thus, all dark bars are above the 'zero' horizontal line. In the second period, in virtually every age group, the change was less than in the first time period (the light bars are lower than the dark bars), and in some cases it was negative (the light bars are below the 'zero' line, indicating that life expectancy actually declined).

32 Figure 2.6 is almost identical to Figure 2.5 (see explanation in note 31), the difference being that instead of comparing life expectancy changes between the two periods by age group, here it is comparing it by different cause of death.

33 These *causal* pathways, the processes that link what epidemiologists refer to as the exposure (in this case whatever has caused the changes to death rates and life expectancy) to the outcome (here, the changes themselves) are discussed in more detail in Chapter 3.

34 This is taken from the 'GHQ-12' (GHQ stands for General Health Questionnaire), which is a well-known and validated measure of 'psychological distress' that is used in population surveys. Responses to 12 questions are summed, with a score of 4 or more denoting psychological distress.

35 Zhang A, Gagné T, Walsh D, Ciancio A, Proto E, McCartney G. Trends in psychological distress in Great Britain, 1991–2019: evidence from three representative surveys. *Journal of Epidemiology and Community Health* 2023; **77**: 468.

36 Walsh D, Wyper GMA, McCartney G. Trends in healthy life expectancy in the age of austerity. *Journal of Epidemiology and Community Health* 2022; **76**: 743.

37 Figure 2.7 shows trends in a common measure of poor mental health

(psychological stress) by year (1991–2019), and by age group 16–34 years (top chart), 35–64 years (middle chart) and 65 years and over (bottom chart). Each line represents the percentage of people in that age group who are deemed to be experiencing psychological distress, based on a score from a survey question (the GHQ-12: a 12 item 'General Health Questionnaire'). Each of the three charts includes data from three separate surveys: Understanding Society (which covers Great Britain), the Scottish Health Survey (which covers Scotland), and the Health Survey for England (which covers England).

38 Figure 2.8 shows trends in Healthy Life Expectancy (HLE) between 1995 and 2019 for Scotland and its 20 per cent most (long-dashed line at the bottom of the chart) and least (short-dashed line at top) socioeconomically deprived populations. HLE is defined as the number of years that would be lived in 'good' or 'very good' health if current mortality and self-rated health data applied for the rest of people's lives. It is derived from a combination of mortality data on how long people are living and surveys of how the population rate their health. The data show that in 1995 people in Scotland were – on average – living around 54 years (53.7 to be precise) in good/very good health, and this had increased to 62.4 years by 2011. However, between 2011 and 2019 it reduced to 60.4 years. In 2019 the HLE in the least deprived areas of Scotland was 70.3 years; in the most deprived areas it was 46.6 years (having declined by 5 years over the decade).

39 Galea S. Compassion in a time of COVID-19. *The Lancet* 2020; **395**: 1897–8.

40 Resnick A, Galea S, Sivashanker K. COVID-19: the painful price of ignoring health inequities. 2020; published online 18 March. https://blogs.bmj.com/bmj/2020/03/18/covid-19-the-painful-price-of-ignoring-health-inequities/.

41 Katikireddi SV, Lal S, Carrol ED, et al. Unequal impact of the COVID-19 crisis on minority ethnic groups: a framework for understanding and addressing inequalities. *Journal of Epidemiology & Community Health* 2021; **75**: 970–4.

42 Bambra C, Lynch J, Smith KE. *The unequal pandemic COVID-19 and health inequalities*. Bristol: Policy Press, 2021.

43 Bambra C, Marmot M. *Expert report for the UK COVID-19 public inquiry. Module 1: health inequalities.* London: UK Covid-19 Public Inquiry, 2023 https://covid19.public-inquiry.uk/documents/inq000195843-expert-report-by-professor-clare-bambra-and-professor-sir-michael-marmot-dated-30-may-2023/.

44 UKHSA. *COVID-19 confirmed deaths in England (to 31 December 2022).* London: UK Health Security Agency, 2023 https://www.gov.uk/government/publications/covid-19-reported-sars-cov-2-deaths-in-england/covid-19-confirmed-deaths-in-england-to-31-december-2022-report.

45 Douglas M, McCartney G, Richardson E, Taulbut M, Craig N. *Population health impacts of the rising cost of living in Scotland: a rapid health impact assessment.* Edinburgh: Public Health Scotland, 2022 https://publichealthscotland.scot/publications/population-health-impacts-of-the-rising-cost-of-living-in-scotland-a-rapid-health-impact-assessment/population-health-impacts-of-the-rising-cost-of-living-in-scotland-a-rapid-health-impact-assessment/.

46 Richardson E, McCartney G, Taulbut M, Douglas M, Craig N. Population mortality impacts of the rising cost of living in Scotland: scenario modelling study. *BMJ Public Health* 2023; **1**: e000097.

47 It should be emphasised that there are a great many different forms of health inequality, pertaining to – for example – ethnicity, gender, age, disability, geography and more. Here we are specifically talking about socioeconomic inequalities.

48 As statisticians and epidemiologists would be quick to point out, these are not only crude definitions, but strictly speaking also inaccurate ones. Although indicators of inequality based on the simple absolute or relative difference between two groups for example, richest vs poorest, social class I vs social class V) do exist, the measures shown here in Figure 2.9 – the Slope Index of Inequality (SII) and the Relative Index of Inequality (RII) – are more sophisticated ones, and are based on the calculation of absolute and relative differences across the whole population (here all five quintiles [20 per cent] of socioeconomic deprivation) not just the two most extreme groups.

49 This often confuses people, and no wonder. But in many periods of time in many countries it's been common for these two forms of inequality to be moving in opposite directions; that is, decreasing absolute inequalities and increasing relative inequalities. It's perhaps easier to explain with a made-up example (one that again will again annoy the statisticians with its crude over-simplicity and ill-informed definitions). Imagine two groups of people, one rich and one poor. Let's say that at the start of a decade the poor group has a mortality rate of 250 (per x thousand population), and the rich group has a mortality rate of 125. This is an absolute difference of 125 (250 minus 125) and a relative difference of 2 (because 250 is two times 125). If, by the end of the decade, the rate in the poor group has decreased to 150, and the rate in the rich group has decreased to 50, then the absolute gap is now 100 (150 minus 50) and the relative gap is 3 (because 150 is 3 times 50). Thus, absolute inequalities have decreased but relative inequalities have increased. And at the heart of this apparent contradiction is that mortality rates have improved over time in both populations, but to a greater extent in the rich group. These contrasting trends have allowed people (particularly politicians) to pick and choose which measures they use as evidence

of the success (or otherwise) of policies. And this is why it's important to be aware of, and include, both types of measure in any analysis of health inequalities.

50 SII = Slope Index of Inequality; RII – Relative Index of Inequality.

51 Figure 2.9 shows trends in absolute mortality inequalities (the Slope Index of Inequality [SII]) and relative mortality inequalities (the Relative Index of Inequality [RII]) for all-cause mortality rates for males in Scotland (top) and England (bottom) between 2001/03 and 2015/17. Both measures are calculated from mortality rates for the five deprivation quintiles of each country. In both Scotland and England absolute inequalities reduced until the early 2010s, but increased thereafter. Relative inequalities generally increased over the whole period shown. An attempt at explaining how these two measures of inequality can be seen – at times – to be going in different directions (one increasing, one decreasing) is included within the worked example in note 49. However, the more important issue here is that since the early 2010s, both these measures of inequality have been increasing in both nations of the UK.

Frances

1 UK Government. *Welfare Reform Act 2012*. London: The Stationery Office, 2012 https://www.legislation.gov.uk/ukpga/2012/5/pdfs/ukpga_20120005_en.pdf.

2 Moffatt S, Lawson S, Patterson R, et al. A qualitative study of the impact of the UK 'bedroom tax'. *Journal of Public Health* 2016; **38**: 197–205.

3 Butler P, Siddique H. The bedroom tax explained. *The Guardian*. 2016; published online 27 Jan. https://www.theguardian.com/society/2016/jan/27/the-bedroom-tax-explained.

4 Andrew E, Croal P. *Average household income, UK: financial year ending 2022*. London: Office for National Statistics, 2023 https://www.ons.gov.uk/peoplepopulationandcommunity/personalandhouseholdfinances/incomeandwealth/bulletins/householddisposableincomeandinequality/financialyearending2022.

5 When the legislation was introduced, the median income of social housing tenants in the UK – two-thirds of whom had no savings – was less than £9,000 per annum. The household income figure for the whole population at the time was around £25,000.

6 The policy particularly affected social housing tenants in England. In Scotland the Scottish Government mitigated the effect of the policy by compensating affected tenants with additional money ('discretional housing payments'), and similar actions were taken in Wales and Northern Ireland.

7   Scottish Government. *Discretionary housing payments to mitigate the bedroom tax in Scotland. FOI release.* Edinburgh: Scottish Government https://www.gov.scot/publications/foi-202000014853.

8   Welsh Government. *Mitigating the impact of the UK Government's welfare reforms.* Cardiff: Welsh Government, 2015 https://www.gov.wales/sites/default/files/publications/2019-05/mitigating-the-impact-of-the-uk-governments-welfare-reforms.pdf.

9   Northern Ireland Housing Executive. *Social sector size criteria – bedroom tax.* Northern Ireland Housing Executive https://www.nihe.gov.uk/housing-help/housing-benefit/social-sector-size-criteria-(bedroom-tax).

10 The UK government prefers to describe it as the 'the removal of the spare room subsidy'.

11 Department for Work and Pensions. *Evaluation of removal of the spare room subsidy – final report.* London: Department for Work and Pensions, 2015 https://assets.publishing.service.gov.uk/government/uploads/system/uploads/attachment_data/file/506407/rsrs-evaluation.pdf.

12 Waddington M. Liverpool mum suicide attempt as she struggled to cope with bedroom tax. *Liverpool Echo.* 2013; published online 8 June. https://www.liverpoolecho.co.uk/news/liverpool-news/liverpool-mum-suicide-attempt-struggled-4279433.

13 BBC News. Stephanie Bottrill suicide note blames government. *BBC.* 2013; published online 13 May. https://www.bbc.co.uk/news/uk-england-birmingham-22500009.

14 Morris S. Woman worried about bedroom tax killed herself, coroner finds. *The Guardian.* 2014; published online 12 Aug. https://www.theguardian.com/society/2014/aug/12/stephanie-bottrill-worried-bedroom-tax-committed-suicide-coroner.

15 Grieving mum found hanged near bedroom tax eviction letter had written poverty plea to David Cameron. *Daily Mirror.* 2016; published online 22 Jan. https://www.mirror.co.uk/news/uk-news/grieving-mum-found-hanged-near-7223683.

Chapter 3

1   McCormack C. *The wee yellow butterfly.* Glendaruel: Argyll Publishing, 2009.

2   McCartney G, Walsh D, Fenton L, Devine R. *Resetting the course for population health.* Glasgow: Glasgow Centre for Population Health and the University of Glasgow, 2022.

3   Osborne G. *Speech by the Chancellor of the Exchequer, Rt Hon George Osborne MP, at the Queen's Speech economy debate.* London: House of Commons, 2010 https://www.gov.uk/government/speeches/speech-by-the-chancellor-of-the-exchequer-rt-hon-george-osborne-mp-at-the-queens-speech-economy-debate.

4　David Cameron's Conservative conference speech. *BBC News*. 2011; published online 5 Oct. https://www.bbc.co.uk/news/uk-politics-15189614.

5　Peston R. Is Cameron more Thatcher than Thatcher? *BBC News*. 2014; published online 1 Oct. https://www.bbc.co.uk/news/business-29449222.

6　Blyth M. *Austerity: the history of a dangerous idea*. Cary, NC: Oxford University Press, 2013.

7　Reeves A, Basu S, McKee M, Marmot M, Stuckler D. Austere or not? UK Coalition government budgets and health inequalities. *Journal of the Royal Society of Medicine* 2013; **106**: 432–6.

8　Stiglitz J. Austerity has been an utter disaster for the eurozone. *The Guardian*. 2014; published online 1 Oct. https://www.theguardian.com/business/2014/oct/01/austerity-eurozone-disaster-joseph-stiglitz.

9　Inman P, Traynor I, Rushe D. UK austerity v US stimulus: divide deepens as eurozone cuts continue. *The Guardian*. 2012; published online 14 Feb. https://www.theguardian.com/business/2012/feb/14/austerity-stimulus-divide-eurozone-cuts.

10　Calvert Jump R, Michell J, Meadway J, Nascimento N. *The macroeconomics of austerity*. London: Progressive Economy Forum, 2023.

11　*IMF Datamapper: GDP 2023*. New York: International Monetary Fund (IMF), 2023. https://www.imf.org/external/datamapper/PPPGDP@WEO/OEMDC/ADVEC/WEOWORLD.

12　This applies to England only; in Scotland, Wales and Northern Ireland, local public health activities come under the control of the National Health Service, not local government.

13　It is worth pointing out that local authorities have statutory responsibilities to deliver key services. Thus, they have both 'mandatory' and 'discretionary' functions. The analyses by Mia Gray and Anna Barford (2018) show that there is often a blurred line between these two types of functions: for example, in England services for 'at risk' children are mandatory, while the provision of youth centres for low-income youths are discretionary – yet youth centres seek to particularly help 'at risk' children. Even more importantly, their analyses show that while discretionary services often received greater cuts, both types of services (including those deemed mandatory) have been cut to a huge degree, and have limited local authorities' abilities to deliver them.

14　At the time of writing, this is now called the Department for Levelling Up, Housing and Communities.

15　This was considerably more than, for example, the c. 25 per cent reduction in funds to the Home Office or the c. 30 per cent reduction in funding of the Department of Environment, Food and Rural Affairs (Gray and Barford, 2018).

16 Gray M, Barford A. The depths of the cuts: the uneven geography of local government austerity. *Cambridge Journal of Regions, Economy and Society* 2018; **11**: 541–63.

17 Note that Gray and Barford's analyses included local government in only Scotland, England and Wales; Northern Ireland was therefore excluded.

18 *Facts on social security*. Geneva: International Labour Office, 2003.

19 Scottish Government. *Welfare Reform (Further Provision) (Scotland) Act 2012: annual report 2017*. Edinburgh: Scottish Government, 2017.

20 Estimates range from around £26 billion (Beatty and Fothergill, 2016 [see note 23]; Beatty and Fothergill, 2018 [see note 22] – although described by the authors as 'probably too low') to £56 billion (Women's Budget Group [De Henau 2017, see note 24]). Suggested 'mid–way' figures of around £37 billion (for example, a separate estimate from the Women's Budget Group (WBG), and one cited by ex–MP Frank Field) may be more appropriate, but we cannot be certain.

21 Beatty C. Personal communication. Sheffield: Sheffield Hallam University, 2022.

22 Beatty C, Fothergill S. Welfare reform in the United Kingdom 2010–16: expectations, outcomes, and local impacts. *Social Policy & Administration* 2018; **52**: 950–68.

23 Beatty C, Fothergill S. *The uneven impact of welfare reform: the financial losses to places and people*. Sheffield: Sheffield Hallam, 2016.

24 De Henau J. *Gender impact of social security spending cuts*. London: Women's Budget Group, 2017 https://wbg.org.uk/wp-content/uploads/2017/03/WBG_briefing_Soc-Security_pre_Budget.pdf.

25 Butler P. Welfare spending for UK's poorest shrinks by £37bn. *The Guardian*, 2018; published online 23 Sept. https://www.theguardian.com/politics/2018/sep/23/welfare-spending-uk-poorest-austerity-frank-field.

26 *2010 to 2015 government policy: welfare reform*. London: Department for Work and Pensions, 2015 https://www.gov.uk/government/publications/2010-to-2015-government-policy-welfare-reform/2010-to-2015-government-policy-welfare-reform.

27 UK Government. *Welfare Reform Act 2012*. London: The Stationery Office, 2012 https://www.legislation.gov.uk/ukpga/2012/5/pdfs/ukpga_20120005_en.pdf.

28 *Welfare Reform and Work Act 2016*. London: UK Government, 2016.

29 *Welfare trends report*. London: Office for Budget Responsibility, 2016 https://obr.uk/docs/dlm_uploads/Welfare-Trends-Report.pdf.

30 Taulbut M, Agbato D, McCartney G. *Working and hurting? Monitoring the health and health inequalities impacts of the economic downturn and changes to the social security system*. Glasgow: NHS Health Scotland, 2018.

31 McCartney G, Myers F, Taulbut M, et al. *Making a bad situation worse? The impact of welfare reform and the economic recession on health and health inequalities in Scotland (baseline report).* Edinburgh: NHS Health Scotland, 2013.

32 *Inflation data for UK.* New York: World Bank, 2023 https://data.worldb ank.org/indicator/FP.CPI.TOTL.ZG?locations=GB.

33 From 2011, the Consumer Price Index (CPI) was used instead of the Retail Price Index (RPI). The former is usually lower than the latter.

34 *Universal Credit isn't working: proposals for reform.* London: House of Lords Economic Affairs Committee, 2020.

35 Fitzpatrick S, Bramley G, Treanor M, et al. *Destitution in the UK 2023.* York: Joseph Rowntree Foundation, 2023.

36 Kennedy S, Hobson F, Mackley A, Kirk-Wade E, Lewis A. Department for Work and Pensions policy on benefit sanctions. London: House of Commons Library, 2022 https://commonslibrary.parliament.uk/resea rch-briefings/cdp-2022-0230/.

37 Webster D. *Briefing: benefit sanctions statistics – May 2023.* London: Child Poverty Action Group, 2023 https://cpag.org.uk/policy-and-campai gns/briefing/david-webster-university-glasgow-briefings-benefit-sanctions.

38 The draft report by the UK government DWP was completed in August 2020; however, the government then refused to publish it. Multiple Freedom of Information requests from David Webster at the University of Glasgow were also refused, resulting in a successful appeal to the UK Information Commissioner. The government was ordered to publish the report, and this finally took place in April 2023.

39 *The impact of benefit sanctions on employment outcomes.* London: Department for Work and Pensions, 2023 https://www.gov.uk/government/ publications/the-impact-of-benefit-sanctions-on-employment-outco mes-draft-report/the-impact-of-benefit-sanctions-on-employment-outcomes.

40 Webster D. *Commentary on the DWP report 'the impact of benefit sanctions on employment outcomes'.* London: Child Poverty Action Group, 2023 https://cpag.org.uk/policy-and-campaigns/briefing/david-webster-uni versity-glasgow-briefings-benefit-sanctions.

41 Scottish Government. *Discretionary housing payments to mitigate the bedroom tax in Scotland. FOI release.* Edinburgh: Scottish Government https:// www.gov.scot/publications/foi-202000014853.

42 Welsh Government. *Mitigating the impact of the UK Government's welfare reforms.* Cardiff: Welsh Government, 2015 https://www.gov.wales/sites/ default/files/publications/2019-05/mitigating-the-impact-of-the-uk-governments-welfare-reforms.pdf.

43 Northern Ireland Housing Executive. *Social sector size criteria – bedroom tax*. Northern Ireland Housing Executive https://www.nihe.gov.uk/housing-help/housing-benefit/social-sector-size-criteria-(bedroom-tax).

44 Note that these changes related to Local Housing Allowance (LHA). LHA is not a separate benefit but, rather, a means of assessing the level of rent eligible for housing benefit to which an applicant may be entitled.

45 Walker P, Butler P. Government under fire over new child tax credit form for rape victims. *The Guardian*. 2017; published online April 6. https://www.theguardian.com/society/2017/apr/06/government-under-fire-over-new-child-tax-credit-form-for-victims.

46 Loopstra R, McKee M, Katikireddi SV, Taylor-Robinson D, Barr B, Stuckler D. Austerity and old-age mortality in England: a longitudinal cross-local area analysis, 2007–2013. *Journal of the Royal Society of Medicine* 2016; **109**: 109–16.

47 *A3/2019 Mixed age couples: changes to entitlement conditions from 15 May 2019*. London: Department for Work and Pensions, 2019 https://www.gov.uk/government/publications/housing-benefit-adjudication-circulars-2019/a32018-mixed-age-couples-changes-to-entitlement-conditions-from-15-may-2019.

48 *The cumulative impact of welfare reform: a national picture*. London: Policy in Practice and Local Government Association, 2017 https://policyinpractice.co.uk/wp-content/uploads/2017/06/The-impact-of-welfare-reform-a-national-picture_summary-report.pdf.

49 Portes J, Reed H. *The cumulative impact of tax and welfare reforms*. Manchester: Equality and Human Rights Commission (EHRC), 2018.

50 Figure 3.1 shows the change in people's income by 2021/22 that has been estimated to have been caused by the social security and related taxation changes introduced (between 2010 and 2018) as part of the UK government austerity policies. The figures are shown as percentages, and broken down into ten groups according to people's income levels – from the 10th of the population with the lowest income (the poorest) to the 10th of the population with the highest income (the richest). While those in the two poorest groups lost between 9 per cent and 9.7 per cent of their income, those in the richest group saw no change to their income at all.

51 According to the 2011 Census, the socioeconomic profiles of ethnic minority groups in England and Scotland were quite different, with many groups much less deprived in Scotland than in England. However, at the time of writing, the results of Scottish 2022 Census are not yet available, and it is possible this situation has altered.

52 Walsh D, Buchanan D, Douglas A, et al. Increasingly diverse: the changing ethnic profiles of Scotland and Glasgow and the implications for population health. *Applied Spatial Analysis and Policy* 2019; **12**: 983–1009.

53 These include impacts such as: the expansion of Universal Credit, which was seen as disincentivising second income earners in a household, most of whom are female; cuts to legal aid/advice, which has had a detrimental impact on females wishing to challenge discriminatory employment practices; and cuts to specific services for young children and in relation to gender-based violence.

54 Hudson-Sharp N, Munro-Lott N, Rolfe H, Runge J. *Impact of welfare reform and welfare-to-work programmes: an evidence review.* Manchester: Equality and Human Rights Commission (EHRC), 2018.

55 Reis S. *The impact of austerity on women in the UK.* London: Women's Budget Group, 2018.

56 Browne J. *The impact of tax and benefit reforms by sex: some simple analysis.* London: Institute of Fiscal Studies, 2011.

57 Keen R, Cracknell R. *Estimating the gender impact of tax and benefits changes.* London: House of Commons Library, 2017.

58 Rafferty A. Gender equality and the impact of recession and austerity in the UK. *Revue de l'OFCE, Presses de Sciences-Po* 2014; **0**: 335–61.

59 Busby N, James G. Regulating work and care relationships in a time of austerity: a legal perspective. In: Lewis S, Anderson D, Lyonette C, Payne N, Wood S, eds. *Work–life balance in times of recession, austerity and beyond.* Abingdon: Routledge, 2016.

60 Hall S, McIntosh K, Neitzert E, et al. *Intersecting inequalities: the impact of austerity on Black and minority ethnic women in the UK.* London: Women's Budget Group, 2017 https://barrowcadbury.org.uk/wp-content/uplo ads/2017/10/Intersecting-Inequalities-October-2017-Full-Report.pdf.

61 A common focus of recent analyses in societal and health inequalities is the issue of intersectionality – multiple aspects of disadvantage (or advantage) operating in combination.

62 Link BG, Phelan JC. McKeown and the idea that social conditions are fundamental causes of disease. *American Journal of Public Health* 2002; **92**: 730–2.

63 McCartney G, Collins C, Mackenzie M. What (or who) causes health inequalities: theories, evidence and implications? *Health Policy* 2013; **113**: 221–7.

64 Commission on the Social Determinants of Health. *Closing the gap in a generation: health equity through action on the social determinants of health.* Geneva: WHO, 2008.

65 Marmot M, Allen J, Goldblatt P, et al. *Fair society, healthy lives: Marmot review report.* London: Institute of Health Equity.

66 Gunasekara FI, Carter K, Blakely T. Change in income and change in self-rated health: systematic review of studies using repeated measures to control for confounding bias. *Social Science & Medicine* 2011; **72**: 193–201.

67 Poverty can be measured in different ways. The Joseph Rowntree Foundation and other organisations recommend the use of 'relative poverty', which is defined as having an income less than 60 per cent of the median income for the population in that year. Thus for any year, people's income is compared with the rest of the population in that same year. In contrast, the official definition of 'absolute poverty' is income below 60 per cent of the country median in one particular year – current publications use 2010/11. This is clearly a very different definition from international measures of absolute poverty, which are more about being unable to achieve basic living standards (food, shelter and so on). As this technical measure of 'absolute poverty' compares everything against income at a fixed point in time, and given that one would normally expect incomes to rise over time, absolute poverty is more likely to improve (even though it is adjusted for inflation) – it is also therefore more likely to be quoted by governments.

68 *UK poverty 2023*. York: Joseph Rowntree Foundation, 2023 https://www.jrf.org.uk/report/uk-poverty-2023.

69 Sosenko F, Bramley G, Bhattacharjee A. Understanding the post–2010 increase in food bank use in England: new quasi–experimental analysis of the role of welfare policy. *BMC Public Health* 2022; **22**: 1363.

70 End of year stats. The Trussell Trust. 2024; published online April. https://www.trusselltrust.org/news–and–blog/latest–stats/end–year–stats/.

71 Figure 3.3 shows the total number of food parcels distributed by the Trussell Trust network in each financial year (running from 1 April to 31 March the following year) between 2010/11 (when around 61,500 parcels were distributed) and 2019/20 (when the figure was just under two million). The figures pre–date the COVID-19 pandemic and the later post-pandemic period of high inflation (cost-of-living crisis), and it should be noted that by 2022/23 the total figure had increased to almost three million (2,986,203). While the increase in the number of food parcels will have been driven to an extent by the increase in the number of food banks which opened (particularly in the early 2010s), that increase in the number of food banks was driven by unmet need in local areas.

72 Most food banks require people to be 'referred' – you can't just turn up. Referrals can be made by Citizens Advice Bureaux, social workers, general practitioners and others.

73 Prayogo E, Chater A, Chapman S, et al. Who uses foodbanks and why? Exploring the impact of financial strain and adverse life events on food insecurity. *Journal of Public Health* 2018; **40**: 676–83.

74 Systematic reviews are comprehensive reviews and syntheses of all the published international evidence for a topic. There are very clear guidelines for how to undertake one, and these need to be followed. Only the most masochistic of researchers actually enjoy doing them.

75 Jenkins RH, Aliabadi S, Vamos EP, et al. The relationship between austerity and food insecurity in the UK: A systematic review. *eClinicalMedicine* 2021; **33**. DOI:10.1016/j.eclinm.2021.100781.

76 Francis-Devine B, Malik X, Danechi S. *Food poverty: households, food banks and free school meals*. London: House of Commons Library, 2023 https://commonslibrary.parliament.uk/research-briefings/cbp-9209/.

77 'Food insecurity' is a (arguably unhelpful and unintuitive) term which in effect means people going hungry: not being able to afford to eat. According to the Trussell Trust, is refers to when people 'have run out of food and been unable to afford more; and/or reduced their meal size, eaten less, gone hungry or lost weight due to a lack of money'.

78 The Trussell Trust. *Hunger in the UK*. Salisbury: The Trussell Trust, 2023 https://www.trusselltrust.org/wp-content/uploads/sites/2/2023/06/2023-Hunger-in-the-UK-policy-briefing.pdf.

79 Loopstra R, Reeves A, Barr B, Taylor-Robinson D, McKee M, Stuckler D. The impact of economic downturns and budget cuts on homelessness claim rates across 323 local authorities in England, 2004–12. *Journal of Public Health* 2016; **38**: 417–25.

80 Dearden L. Conservative austerity policies may have driven homelessness rise, housing secretary admits. *The Independent.* 2018; published online 24 Dec. https://www.independent.co.uk/news/uk/politics/austerity-homeless-crisis-housing-rough-sleeping-conservatives-james-brokenshire-a8698661.html.

81 Copley T. *Homelessness: the visible effect of austerity*. London: London Assembly Labour, 2019 https://www.london.gov.uk/sites/default/files/tom_copley_am_homelessness_-_the_visible_effect_of_austerity.pdf.

82 Thunder J, Bovill RC. *Local authority spending on homelessness: understanding recent trends and their impact*. Middlesex: WPI Economics, 2020 https://wpieconomics.com/site/wp-content/uploads/2019/04/Local-authority-spending-on-homelessness-FULL-FINAL.pdf.

83 Ellis K, Leahy Laughlin D. Youth homelessness in austerity Britain: 'We can't help you, you need to go back home'. *Child & Youth Services* 2021; **42**: 302–17.

84 Boffey D, Helm T. Eric Pickles warns David Cameron of rise in homeless families risk. *Observer.* 2011; published online 2 July. https://www.theguardian.com/politics/2011/jul/02/eric-pickles-david-cameron-40000-homeless.

85 Scott C, Sutherland J, Taylor A. *Affordability of the UK's Eatwell Guide*. London: The Food Foundation, 2018.

86 McEwen BS. Brain on stress: how the social environment gets under the skin. *Proceedings of the National Academy of Sciences 2012;* **109**: 17180–5.

87   McLean J. *Psychological, social and biological determinants of ill health (pSoBid) in Glasgow: a cross-sectional, population-based study – final study report*. Glasgow: Glasgow Centre for Population Health, 2014.

88   Elliott I. *Poverty and mental health: a review to inform the Joseph Rowntree Foundation's anti-poverty strategy*. London: Mental Health Foundation, 2016.

89   Russ TC, Stamatakis E, Hamer M, Starr JM, Kivimäki M, Batty GD. Association between psychological distress and mortality: individual participant pooled analysis of 10 prospective cohort studies. *BMJ* 2012; **345**: e4933.

90   Batty GD, Russ TC, Stamatakis E, Kivimäki M. Psychological distress in relation to site specific cancer mortality: pooling of unpublished data from 16 prospective cohort studies. *BMJ* 2017; **356**: j108.

91   Baker C. *Suicide statistics*. London: House of Commons Library, 2022 https://researchbriefings.files.parliament.uk/documents/CBP-7749/CBP-7749.pdf.

92   Marmot M, Wilkinson R. *Social determinants of health: the solid facts.* 2nd edition. Copenhagen: World Health Organisation, 2003.

93   Marmot M, Wilkinson R. *Social determinants of health, 2nd edition.* Oxford: Oxford Academic, 2005.

94   Dahlgren G, Whitehead M. *European strategies for tackling social inequities in health: levelling up, Part 2*. Copenhagen: WHO Regional Office for Europe, 2007.

95   Evans RG, Stoddart GL. Producing health, consuming health care. In: *Why are some people healthy and others not? The determinants of health of populations*. Berlin and New York: Walter de Gruyter, 1994.

96   Krieger N. *Epidemiology and the people's health. Theory and context.* Oxford: Oxford University Press, 2011.

97   Lee SC, DelPozo-Banos M, Lloyd K, Jones I, Walters JTR, John A. Trends in socioeconomic inequalities in incidence of severe mental illness: a population-based linkage study using primary and secondary care routinely collected data between 2000 and 2017. *Schizophrenia Research* 2023; **260**: 113–22.

98   Barr B, Kinderman P, Whitehead M. Trends in mental health inequalities in England during a period of recession, austerity and welfare reform 2004 to 2013. *Social Science & Medicine* 2015; **147**: 324–31.

99   Reeves A, Clair A, McKee M, Stuckler D. Reductions in the United Kingdom's government housing benefit and symptoms of depression in low-income households. *American Journal of Epidemiology* 2016; **184**: 421–9.

100   Reeves A, Fransham M, Stewart K, Patrick R. Does capping social security harm health? A natural experiment in the UK. *Social Policy & Administration* 2022; **56**: 345–59.

101   Kim C, Teo C, Nielsen A, Chum A. What are the mental health consequences of austerity measures in public housing? A quasi-experimental study. *Journal of Epidemiology and Community Health* 2022; **76**: 730.

102   Cherrie M, Curtis S, Baranyi G, et al. A data linkage study of the effects of the great recession and austerity on antidepressant prescription usage. *European Journal of Public Health* 2021; **31**: 297–303.

103   Wickham S, Bentley L, Rose T, Whitehead M, Taylor-Robinson D, Barr B. Effects on mental health of a UK welfare reform, Universal Credit: a longitudinal controlled study. *The Lancet Public Health* 2020; **5**: e157–64.

104   Fahy K, Alexiou A, Daras K, et al. Mental health impact of cuts to local government spending on cultural, environmental and planning services in England: a longitudinal ecological study. *BMC Public Health* 2023; **23**: 1441.

105   Katikireddi SV, Molaodi OR, Gibson M, Dundas R, Craig P. Effects of restrictions to Income Support on health of lone mothers in the UK: a natural experiment study. *The Lancet Public Health* 2018; **3**: e333–40.

106   Barr B, Taylor-Robinson D, Stuckler D, Loopstra R, Reeves A, Whitehead M. 'First, do no harm': are disability assessments associated with adverse trends in mental health? A longitudinal ecological study. *Journal of Epidemiology and Community Health* 2016; **70**: 339.

107   Simpson J, Albani V, Bell Z, Bambra C, Brown H. Effects of social security policy reforms on mental health and inequalities: a systematic review of observational studies in high-income countries. *Social Science & Medicine* 2021; **272**: 113717.

108   This is the national health improvement agency in Scotland.

109   Richardson E, Fenton L, Parkinson J, et al. The effect of income-based policies on mortality inequalities in Scotland: a modelling study. *The Lancet Public Health* 2020; **5**: e150–6.

110   Seaman R, Walsh D, Beatty C, McCartney G, Dundas R. Social security cuts and life expectancy: a longitudinal analysis of local authorities in England, Scotland and Wales. *Journal of Epidemiology and Community Health* 2023; **78**: jech-2023-220328.

111   This is clearly a much lower estimate of the number of excess deaths than was quoted in Chapters 1 and 2. That is for three reasons: the lower figure is for a much shorter time period (2010/11 to 2014/15); it is in relation to funding cuts to only three specific areas (social care, healthcare and public health) and so therefore ignores both wider local government funding cuts and also, importantly, cuts to social security; and it is for England only.

112   Martin S, Longo F, Lomas J, Claxton K. Causal impact of social care, public health and healthcare expenditure on mortality in England: cross-sectional evidence for 2013/2014. *BMJ Open* 2021; **11**: e046417.

113 Alexiou A, Fahy K, Mason K, et al. Local government funding and life expectancy in England: a longitudinal ecological study. *The Lancet Public Health* 2021; **6**: e641–7.

114 Watkins J, Wulaningsih W, Da Zhou C, et al. Effects of health and social care spending constraints on mortality in England: a time trend analysis. *BMJ Open* 2017; **7**: e017722.

115 Maynard A. Shrinking the state: the fate of the NHS and social care. *Journal of the Royal Society of Medicine* 2017; **110**: 49–51.

116 Robertson R, Wenzel L, Thompson J, Charles A. *NHS financial pressures: how are they affecting patient care?* London: King's Fund, 2017.

117 Merry L, Gainsbury S. What was austerity's toll on the NHS before the pandemic? *Nuffield Trust.* 2023; published online 21 June. https://www.nuffieldtrust.org.uk/news-item/what-was-austeritys-toll-on-the-nhs-before-the-pandemic.

118 Stokes J, Bower P, Guthrie B, et al. Cuts to local government spending, multimorbidity and health-related quality of life: a longitudinal ecological study in England. *The Lancet Regional Health – Europe* 2022; **19**. DOI:10.1016/j.lanepe.2022.100436.

119 Jenkins R, Vamos EP, Mason KE, et al. Local area public sector spending and nutritional anaemia hospital admissions in England: a longitudinal ecological study. *BMJ Open* 2022; **12**: e059739.

120 Although this study showed an association between service cuts and the number of people accessing and completing treatment, it did not – unlike other similar studies – show an association between cuts and mortality. However, the paper urges cautious interpretation of the latter negative result, citing methodological and other limitations as possible explanations.

121 Roscoe S, Pryce R, Buykx P, Gavens L, Meier PS. Is disinvestment from alcohol and drug treatment services associated with treatment access, completions and related harm? An analysis of English expenditure and outcomes data. *Drug and Alcohol Review* 2022; **41**: 54–61.

122 Friebel R, Yoo KJ, Maynou L. Opioid abuse and austerity: evidence on health service use and mortality in England. *Social Science & Medicine* 2022; **298**: 114511.

123 Note that although a relationship was demonstrated between cuts and drug-related mortality, the same was not true for alcohol-related deaths.

124 Alexiou A, Mason K, Fahy K, Taylor-Robinson D, Barr B. Assessing the impact of funding cuts to local housing services on drug and alcohol related mortality: a longitudinal study using area-level data in England. *International Journal of Housing Policy* 2023; **23**: 362–80.

125 Koltai J, McKee M, Stuckler D. Association between disability-related budget reductions and increasing drug-related mortality across local authorities in Great Britain. *Social Science & Medicine* 2021; **284**: 114225.

126 Walsh D, Dundas R, McCartney G, Gibson M, Seaman R. Bearing the burden of austerity: how do changing mortality rates in the UK compare between men and women? *Journal of Epidemiology and Community Health* 2022; **76**: 1027.

127 Bennett JE, Pearson-Stuttard J, Kontis V, Capewell S, Wolfe I, Ezzati M. Contributions of diseases and injuries to widening life expectancy inequalities in England from 2001 to 2016: a population-based analysis of vital registration data. *The Lancet Public Health* 2018; **3**: e586–97.

128 Rashid T, Bennett JE, Paciorek CJ, et al. Life expectancy and risk of death in 6791 communities in England from 2002 to 2019: high-resolution spatiotemporal analysis of civil registration data. *The Lancet Public Health* 2021; **6**: e805–16.

129 Currie J, Boyce T, Evans L, et al. Life expectancy inequalities in Wales before COVID-19: an exploration of current contributions by age and cause of death and changes between 2002 and 2018. *Public Health* 2021; **193**: 48–56.

130 Thomson RM, Niedzwiedz CL, Katikireddi SV. Trends in gender and socioeconomic inequalities in mental health following the great recession and subsequent austerity policies: a repeat cross-sectional analysis of the health surveys for England. *BMJ Open* 2018; **8**: e022924.

131 Zhang A, Gagné T, Walsh D, Ciancio A, Proto E, McCartney G. Trends in psychological distress in Great Britain, 1991–2019: evidence from three representative surveys. *Journal of Epidemiology and Community Health* 2023; **77**: 468.

132 Rajmil L, Hjern A, Spencer N, Taylor-Robinson D, Gunnlaugsson G, Raat H. Austerity policy and child health in European countries: a systematic literature review. *BMC Public Health* 2020; **20**: 564.

133 de Mendonça ELSS, de Lima Macêna M, Bueno NB, de Oliveira ACM, Mello CS. Premature birth, low birth weight, small for gestational age and chronic non-communicable diseases in adult life: a systematic review with meta-analysis. *Early Human Development* 2020; **149**: 105154.

134 De Mola CL, De França GVA, de Avila Quevedo L, Horta BL. Low birth weight, preterm birth and small for gestational age association with adult depression: systematic review and meta-analysis. *The British Journal of Psychiatry* 2014; **205**: 340–7.

135 Black SE, Devereux PJ, Salvanes KG. From the cradle to the labor market? The effect of birth weight on adult outcomes. *The Quarterly Journal of Economics* 2007; **122**: 409–39.

136 Blumenshine P, Egerter S, Barclay CJ, Cubbin C, Braveman PA. Socioeconomic disparities in adverse birth outcomes: a systematic review. *American Journal of Preventive Medicine* 2010; **39**: 263–72.

137 Hobel CJ, Goldstein A, Barrett ES. Psychosocial stress and pregnancy outcome. *Clinical Obstetrics and Gynecology* 2008; **51**. https://journals.lww.com/clinicalobgyn/fulltext/2008/06000/psychosocial_stress_and_pregnancy_outcome.17.aspx.

138 Lima SAM, El Dib RP, Rodrigues MRK, et al. Is the risk of low birth weight or preterm labor greater when maternal stress is experienced during pregnancy? A systematic review and meta-analysis of cohort studies. *PLOS ONE* 2018; **13**: e0200594.

139 Watson R, Walsh D, Scott S, Carruthers J, Fenton L, Moore E. Is the period of austerity in the UK associated with increased rates of adverse birth outcomes? (Forthcoming).

140 Figure 3.4 shows trends in the percentage of all live births that were of low birthweight (using the standard definition of less than 2,500g) in Scotland between 1998 and 2019. The solid line in the middle represents all Scotland; the short-dashed line births in the 20 per cent most deprived areas; and the long-dashed line births in the 20 per cent least deprived areas.

141 Sure Start centres were set up to provide a wide range of services to help mothers and children, including: early learning and childcare; support and advice on parenting; child and family health services (for example, antenatal/postnatal support, breastfeeding support, smoking cessation support, nutritional advice); and more.

142 Mason KE, Alexiou A, Bennett DL, Summerbell C, Barr B, Taylor-Robinson D. Impact of cuts to local government spending on Sure Start children's centres on childhood obesity in England: a longitudinal ecological study. *Journal of Epidemiology and Community Health* 2021; **75**: 860.

143 Walsh D, McCartney G, Smith M, Armour G. Relationship between childhood socioeconomic position and adverse childhood experiences (ACEs): a systematic review. *Journal of Epidemiology and Community Health* 2019; **73**: 1087.

144 *Child poverty: a short evidence briefing*. Glasgow: Scottish Public Health Observatory (ScotPHO), NHS Health Scotland, 2018.

145 Childhood obesity: a short evidence briefing. Glasgow: Scottish Public Health Observatory (ScotPHO), NHS Health Scotland, 2018.

146 Cheetham M, Moffatt S, Addison M, Wiseman A. Impact of Universal Credit in north east England: a qualitative study of claimants and support staff. *BMJ Open* 2019; **9**: e029611.

147 Cheetham M, Gibson M, Morris S, Bambra C, Craig P. OP26 The mental health effects of universal credit: qualitative findings from a mixed methods study. *Journal of Epidemiology and Community Health* 2023; **77**: A13.

148 Smith DM. Austerity, health and public safety in low-income neighborhoods: grassroots responses to the decline of local services in southeast England. *Journal of Urban Health* 2023; **100**: 1224–33.

149 Power M, Pybus KJ, Pickett KE, Doherty B. 'The reality is that on Universal Credit I cannot provide the recommended amount of fresh fruit and vegetables per day for my children': moving from a behavioural to a systemic understanding of food practices. *Emerald Open Research* 2023; **1**. DOI: 10.1108/EOR-10-2023-0007.

150 Douglas F, Sapko J, Kiezebrink K, Kyle J. Resourcefulness, desperation, shame, gratitude and powerlessness: common themes emerging from a study of food bank use in northeast Scotland. *AIMS Public Health* 2015; **2**: 297–317.

151 McGrath L, Griffin V, Mundy E. *The psychological impact of austerity*. London: Psychologists Against Austerity, 2015 https://psychchange. org/uploads/9/7/9/7/97971280/paa_briefing_paper.pdf.

152 Mattheys K, Warren J, Bambra C. 'Treading in sand': a qualitative study of the impact of austerity on inequalities in mental health. *Social Policy & Administration* 2018; **52**: 1275–89.

153 Dickinson A, Wills W. Meals on wheels services and the food security of older people. *Health & Social Care in the Community* 2022; **30**: e6699–707.

154 Ploetner C, Telford M, Brækkan K, et al. Understanding and improving the experience of claiming social security for mental health problems in the west of Scotland: a participatory social welfare study. *Journal of Community Psychology* 2020; **48**: 675–92.

155 Barnes MC, Gunnell D, Davies R, et al. Understanding vulnerability to self-harm in times of economic hardship and austerity: a qualitative study. *BMJ Open* 2016; **6**: e010131.

156 Note that Figure 2.6 in the previous chapter showed separate data for causes of death such as ischaemic heart disease and cerebrovascular disease (stroke) – these are part of the broader CVD grouping.

157 Between 2016 and 2019, only 7 per cent of female deaths aged 0–64 years living in the 20 per cent most socioeconomically deprived neighbourhoods of Glasgow were from ischaemic heart disease (IHD) (the largest single category of CVD). This compares with 28 per cent, 16 per cent, 9 per cent for cancer, drugs-related causes and respiratory conditions, respectively (and 27 per cent for 'other' causes). Previous figures for IHD were 12 per cent in 2001–04 and 8 per cent in 2009–11. The equivalent figures for the 20 per cent most deprived areas of Scotland (rather than just Glasgow) are almost identical. Thus deaths from CVD (or at least IHD) are not a major contributory factor to the increased death rates that have been seen for this group of the population.

158 Authors' analyses of National Records for Scotland mortality and population data, 2023.

159 Marmot M, Wilkinson R. Social patterning of individual health behaviours: the case of cigarette smoking. In: *Social determinants of health*. Oxford: Oxford Academic, 2005.

160 Lynch EB. Uncovering the mechanisms underlying the social patterning of diabetes. *eClinicalMedicine* 2020; **19**. DOI:10.1016/j.eclinm.2020.100273.

161 Butland B, Jebb S, Kopelman P, et al. *Tackling obesities: future choices – project report*. London: Foresight, UK Government, 2007.

162 McDowell I. From risk factors to explanation in public health. *Journal of Public Health* 2008; **30**: 219–23.

163 Marmot M. Inclusion health: addressing the causes of the causes. *The Lancet* 2018; **391**: 186–8.

164 Ramsay J, Minton J, Fischbacher C, et al. How have changes in death by cause and age group contributed to the recent stalling of life expectancy gains in Scotland? Comparative decomposition analysis of mortality data, 2000–2002 to 2015–2017. *BMJ Open* 2020; **10**: e036529.

165 *A review of recent trends in mortality in England*. London: Public Health England, 2018.

166 As we mention in the story of Ellen later in the book, the causes of Scotland's higher rates of drug-related deaths are well understood in the research community and, alongside austerity, include factors as diverse as: an ageing cohort of vulnerable drug users experiencing illness and disease; relative affordability of drugs; sophisticated supply mechanisms; and the different types of drugs that have been on the market in different time periods. As this chapter has discussed, the two elements of austerity that are relevant are cuts to services (for example, addiction services) and cuts to individual incomes (social security). With regard to the former, the situation in Scotland is more complex than in England, as any cuts to services have had to be implemented via the devolved government (rather than directly, as occurred in England). And it has been suggested in some quarters than the manner in which those cuts were implemented was different, and more harmful, in Scotland (see reference 149). However, the evidence for this is currently unclear, and further research is required to unpick and better understand the impacts of these different aspects of austerity on the increase in deaths since 2010.

167 McPhee I, Sheridan B. AUDIT Scotland 10 years on: explaining how funding decisions link to increased risk for drug related deaths among the poor. *Drugs and Alcohol Today* 2020; **20**: 313–22.

168 Walsh D, McCartney G. *Changing mortality rates in Scotland and the UK: an updated summary.* Glasgow: Glasgow Centre for Population Health, 2023 https://www.gcph.co.uk/assets/0000/9348/Changing_mortality_rates_in_Scotland_and_the_UK_-_an_updated_summary_FINAL.pdf.

169 Figure 3.5 shows trends in age-standardised mortality rates for 'drug-related poisonings' between 1981 and 2021 for Scotland as a whole (solid line), and for people living in the 20 per cent most deprived (short-dashed line) and the 20 per cent least deprived (long-dashed line) areas of the country. Note that this definition of drug-related poisonings used in here (and in different journal articles) is broader and less accurate than that used in official government agency reports on drugs related deaths. However, the trends in both measures are very similar.

170 *Dementia and Alzheimer's disease deaths including comorbidities, England and Wales: 2019 registrations.* London: Office for National Statistics, 2020 https://www.ons.gov.uk/peoplepopulationandcommunity/birthsdeathsandmarriages/deaths/bulletins/dementiaandalzheimersdiseasedeathsincludingcomorbiditiesenglandandwales/2019registrations.

171 Hiam L, Dorling D, Harrison D, McKee M. What caused the spike in mortality in England and Wales in January 2015? *Journal of the Royal Society of Medicine* 2017; **110**: 131–7.

172 Ahmad S, Carey IM, Harris T, Cook DG, DeWilde S, Strachan DP. The rising tide of dementia deaths: triangulation of data from three routine data sources using the Clinical Practice Research Datalink. *BMC Geriatrics* 2021; **21**: 375.

173 Gao L, Calloway R, Zhao E, Brayne C, Matthews FE, Medical Research Council Cognitive Function and Ageing Collaboration. Accuracy of death certification of dementia in population-based samples of older people: analysis over time. *Age and Ageing* 2018; **47**: 589–94.

174 The software in question applied International Classification of Diseases (ICD10) diagnostic codes to death certificates (ICD10 is a coding system in which every disease has an alpha-numeric code). The software was updated in England in 2011 and 2014, and in Scotland in 2017.

175 *Using ONS mortality data – taking account of changes to cause of death coding from 2014.* London: Public Health England, 2018.

176 *Deaths registered in England and Wales, 2019.* London: Office for National Statistics, 2020.

177 Matthews FE, Stephan BCM, Robinson L, et al. A two decade dementia incidence comparison from the Cognitive Function and Ageing Studies I and II. *Nature Communications* 2016; **7**: 11398.

178 Ahmadi-Abhari S, Guzman-Castillo M, Bandosz P, et al. Temporal trend in dementia incidence since 2002 and projections for prevalence in England and Wales to 2040: modelling study. *BMJ* 2017; **358**: j2856.

179 Newton J. Re: Sharp spike in deaths in England and Wales needs investigating, says public health expert. *BMJ* 2016; **352**: i981.

180 Newton J, Baker A, Fitzpatrick J, Ege F. What's happening with mortality rates in England? 2017; published online 20 July. https://ukhsa.blog.gov.uk/2017/07/20/whats-happening-with-mortality-rates-in-england/.

181 Baker A, Ege F, Fitzpatrick J, Newton J. Response to articles on mortality in England and Wales. *Journal of the Royal Society of Medicine* 2018; **111**: 40–1.

182 Hiam L, Dorling D, McKee M. Austerity, not influenza, caused the UK's health to deteriorate. Let's not make the same mistake again. *Journal of Epidemiology and Community Health* 2021; **75**: 312.

183 Hiam L, Dorling D, McKee M. When experts disagree: interviews with public health experts on health outcomes in the UK 2010–2020. *Public Health* 2023; **214**: 96–105.

184 Walsh D, Tod E, McCartney G, Levin KA. How much of the stalled mortality trends in Scotland and England can be attributed to obesity? *BMJ Open* 2022; **12**: e067310.

185 Epidemiologists would argue that the true percentage that is not explained by obesity is much higher because causal explanations add up to much more than 100 per cent (as several causes can be necessary for an outcome to occur).

186 Razum O. Migrant mortality, healthy migrant effect. In: *Encyclopedia of public health*. New York: Springer, 2008.

187 Walsh D, McCartney G, Minton J, Parkinson J, Shipton D, Whyte B. Deaths from 'diseases of despair' in Britain: comparing suicide, alcohol-related and drug-related mortality for birth cohorts in Scotland, England and Wales, and selected cities. *Journal of Epidemiology and Community Health* 2021; **75**: 1195.

188 Garthwaite K. Fear of the brown envelope: exploring welfare reform with long-term sickness benefits recipients. *Social Policy & Administration* 2014; **48**: 782–98.

189 Garthwaite K, Bambra C. 'How the other half live': lay perspectives on health inequalities in an age of austerity. *Social Science & Medicine* 2017; **187**: 268–75.

190 Milton S, Buckner S, Salway S, Powell K, Moffatt S, Green J. Understanding welfare conditionality in the context of a generational habitus: a qualitative study of older citizens in England. *Journal of Aging Studies* 2015; **34**: 113–22.

191 Hall SM, Pimlott-Wilson H, Horton J. *Austerity across Europe: lived experiences of economic crises*. Abingdon: Routledge, 2022.

192   *Visit to the United Kingdom of Great Britain and Northern Ireland: report of the Special Rapporteur on extreme poverty and human rights.* New York: United Nations (UN) Human Rights Council, 2019.

193   *Levelling up the United Kingdom.* London: UK Government, 2022 https://www.gov.uk/government/publications/levelling-up-the-united-kingdom.

Paul

1   Paul's story is adapted from Frances Ryan's book (*Crippled: austerity and the demonization of disabled people*) with permission and grateful thanks.

2   Ryan F. *Crippled: austerity and the demonization of disabled people.* London: Verso, 2019.

3   Kim N, Jacobson M. Comparison of catastrophic out-of-pocket medical expenditure among older adults in the United States and South Korea: what affects the apparent difference? *BMC Health Services Research* 2022; **22**: 1202.

4   Glied SA, Zhu B. *Catastrophic out-of-pocket health care costs: a problem mainly for middle-income Americans with employer coverage.* New York: The Commonwealth Fund, 2020.

5   Strand EB, Nacul L, Mengshoel AM, et al. Myalgic encephalomyelitis/chronic fatigue syndrome (ME/CFS): investigating care practices pointed out to disparities in diagnosis and treatment across European Union. *PLOS ONE* 2019; **14**: e0225995.

6   Gray M, Barford A. The depths of the cuts: the uneven geography of local government austerity. *Cambridge Journal of Regions, Economy and Society* 2018; **11**: 541–63.

7   Alexiou A, Fahy K, Mason K, et al. Local government funding and life expectancy in England: a longitudinal ecological study. *The Lancet Public Health* 2021; **6**: e641–7.

8   Gillespie T, Hardy K, Watt P. Surplus to the city: austerity urbanism, displacement and 'letting die'. *Environment and Planning A* 2021; **53**: 1713–29.

9   Johns M. *10 years of austerity: eroding resilience in the North.* Manchester and Newcastle: IPPR North, 2020 https://www.ippr.org/files/2020-06/10-years-of-austerity.pdf.

10 Alexiou A, Mason K, Fahy K, Taylor-Robinson D, Barr B. Assessing the impact of funding cuts to local housing services on drug and alcohol related mortality: a longitudinal study using area-level data in England. *International Journal of Housing Policy* 2023; **23**: 362–80.

Chapter 4

1   Fitzgerald P. *The gate of angels.* London: Harper Perennial, 1990.

2   Blyth M. *Austerity: the history of a dangerous idea.* Cary, NC: Oxford University Press, 2013.

3   McCartney G, McMaster R, Shipton D, Harding O, Hearty W. Glossary: economics and health. *Journal of Epidemiology and Community Health* 2022; **76**: 518.

4   Mark Blyth (2013, p 2) defines austerity as a 'form of voluntary deflation in which the economy adjusts through the reduction of wages, prices, and public spending to restore competitiveness, which is (supposedly) best achieved by cutting the state's budget, debts, and deficits'. Thus the definitions of austerity used by economists are a little more sophisticated than that provided here. Essentially, it is a policy approach that assumes that government debt and government deficits harm economic growth, and policies which reduce debt and deficits are an effective way of increasing economic growth, even during economic downturns. Measures of austerity try to isolate the impacts of deliberate policy changes from the so-called 'automatic stabilisers' in the economy, which are the increases in spending on social security benefits and decreases in tax revenues that occur during recessions (and vice versa).

5   McCartney G, Fenton L, Minton J, et al. Is austerity responsible for the recent change in mortality trends across high-income nations? A protocol for an observational study. *BMJ Open* 2020; **10**: e034832.

6   Whiteside H, McBride S, Evans B. *Varieties of austerity*. Bristol: Bristol University Press, 2021.

7   Farnsworth K, Irving Z. Varieties of crisis, varieties of austerity: social policy in challenging times. *Journal of Poverty and Social Justice* 2012; **20**: 133–47.

8   The two most sophisticated measures of austerity – the Cyclically-Adjusted Primary Balance, and the Alesina-Ardagna Fiscal Index – focus on year-to-year changes in the fiscal balance of governments, and as a result the trends in these measures can be unstable over time and difficult to interpret.

9   McCartney G, McMaster R, Popham F, Dundas R, Walsh D. Is austerity a cause of slower improvements in mortality in high-income countries? A panel analysis. *Social Science & Medicine* 2022; **313**: 115397.

10   Ho JY, Hendi AS. Recent trends in life expectancy across high income countries: retrospective observational study. *BMJ* 2018; **362**: k2562.

11   Fenton L, Minton J, Ramsay J, et al. Recent adverse mortality trends in Scotland: comparison with other high-income countries. *BMJ Open* 2019; **9**: e029936.

12   *A review of recent trends in mortality in England*. London: Public Health England, 2018.

13   Rajmil L, Fernández de Sanmamed M-J. Austerity policies and mortality rates in European countries, 2011–2015. *American Journal of Public Health* 2019; **109**: 768–70.

14 Antonakakis N, Collins A. The impact of fiscal austerity on suicide mortality: evidence across the 'eurozone periphery'. *Social Science & Medicine* 2015; **145**: 63–78.

15 Toffolutti V, Suhrcke M. Does austerity really kill? *Economics & Human Biology* 2019; **33**: 211–23.

16 Osborne G. George Osborne's speech to the Conservative party conference in full. *The Guardian*. 2010; published online 4 Oct. https://www.theguardian.com/politics/2010/oct/04/george-osborne-speech-conservative-conference.

17 Munafò MR, Davey Smith G. Repeating experiments is not enough. *Nature* 2018; **553**: 399–401.

18 Lawlor DA, Tilling K, Davey Smith G. Triangulation in aetiological epidemiology. *International Journal of Epidemiology* 2016; **45**: 1866–86.

19 As expressed by Penelope Fitzgerald in *The Gate of Angels*: 'If they don't depend on true evidence, scientists are no better than gossips.'

20 Reinhart CM, Rogoff K. *This time is different: eight centuries of financial folly*. Princeton: Princeton University Press, 2011.

21 Alesina A, Favero C, Giavazzi F. *Austerity: when it works and when it doesn't*. Princeton: Princeton University Press, 2019.

22 Mirowski P, Plehwe D. *The road from Mont Pelerin: the making of the neoliberal thought collective*. Cambridge, MA: Harvard University Press, 2015.

23 Friel S, Townsend B, Fisher M, Harris P, Freeman T, Baum F. Power and the people's health. *Social Science & Medicine* 2021; **282**: 114173.

24 McCartney G, Dickie E, Escobar O, Collins C. Health inequalities, fundamental causes and power: towards the practice of good theory. *Sociology of Health & Illness* 2021; **43**: 20–39.

25 Popay J, Whitehead M, Ponsford R, Egan M, Mead R. Power, control, communities and health inequalities I: theories, concepts and analytical frameworks. *Health Promotion International* 2021; **36**: 1253–63.

26 Figure 4.3 shows the years in which austerity was implemented in Australia, Germany, the Netherlands and the US, between 2010 and 2019. Where the black bars are below the horizontal zero line, this indicates years and countries where there was a reduction in government spending as a percentage of the size of the economy. It shows that Australia had a reduction in government spending in 2010, 2011 and 2017. Germany had a very substantial reduction in spending in 2011, with smaller reductions in 2012 and 2014. The Netherlands consistently reduced government spending between 2011 and 2018. Finally, the US reduced government spending every year between 2010 and 2015.

27 Raleigh VS. Stalling life expectancy in the UK. *BMJ* 2018; **362**: k4050.

28 Saltkjel T, Ingelsrud MH, Dahl E, Halvorsen K. A fuzzy set approach to economic crisis, austerity and public health. Part II: How are configurations of crisis and austerity related to changes in population health across Europe? *Scandinavian Journal of Public Health* 2017; **45**: 48–55.

29 Saltkjel T, Ingelsrud MH, Dahl E, Halvorsen K. A fuzzy set approach to economic crisis, austerity and public health. Part II: How are configurations of crisis and austerity related to changes in population health across Europe? *Scandinavian Journal of Public Health* 2017; **45**: 48–55.

30 Chambers M. Germany to return to austerity after coronavirus crisis – minister. Reuters. 2020; published online 24 March. https://www.reuters.com/article/us-health-coronavirus-germany-altmaier/germany-to-return-to-austerity-after-coronavirus-crisis-minister-idUSKBN21B0QN.

31 Aukerman MJ. Discrimination in Germany: a call for minority rights. *Netherlands Quarterly of Human Rights* 1995; **13**: 237–57.

32 Weinmann M. Barriers to naturalization: how dual citizenship restrictions impede full membership. *International Migration* 2022; **60**: 237–51.

33 Overmans T, Timm-Arnold K-P. Managing austerity: comparing municipal austerity plans in the Netherlands and North Rhine-Westphalia. *Public Management Review* 2016; **18**: 1043–62.

34 Gschwind L, Ratzmann N, Beste J. Protected against all odds? A mixed-methods study on the risk of welfare sanctions for immigrants in Germany. *Social Policy & Administration* 2022; **56**: 502–17.

35 Lampert T, Hoebel J, Kroll LE. Social differences in mortality and life expectancy in Germany. Current situation and trends. *Journal of Health Monitoring* 2019; **4**: 3–14.

36 Nowossadeck E, von der Lippe E, Lampert T. Developments in life expectancy in Germany. Current situation and trends. *Journal of Health Monitoring* 2019; **4**: 38–45.

37 Jasilionis D, van Raalte AA, Klüsener S, Grigoriev P. The underwhelming German life expectancy. *European Journal of Epidemiology* 2023; **38**: 839–50.

38 Baldus S, Lauterbach K. Prevention-centered health care in Germany: a nation in need to turn the tide. *European Journal of Epidemiology* 2023; **38**: 835–7.

39 Sobel M. Germany's curious austerity debate. *OMFIF*. 2021; published online 25 May. https://www.omfif.org/2021/05/germanys-curious-austerity-debate/.

40 McCartney G, Hearty W, Arnot J, Popham F, Cumbers A, McMaster R. Impact of political economy on population health: a systematic review of reviews. *American Journal of Public Health* 2019; **109**: e1–12.

41 Beckfield J, Krieger N. Epi + demos + cracy: linking political systems and priorities to the magnitude of health inequities – evidence, gaps, and a research agenda. *Epidemiologic Reviews* 2009; **31**: 152–77.

42 Lopez AD, Adair T. Slower increase in life expectancy in Australia than in other high income countries: the contributions of age and cause of death. *Medical Journal of Australia* 2019; **210**: 403–9.

43 Bauman AE. Interpreting the 'league tables of death': advance Australia backwards? *Medical Journal of Australia* 2019; **210**: 400–1.

44 Western M, Baxter J, Pakulski J, et al. Neoliberalism, inequality and politics: the changing face of Australia. *Australian Journal of Social Issues* 2007; **42**: 401–18.

45 Beeson M, Firth A. Neoliberalism as a political rationality: Australian public policy since the 1980s. *Journal of Sociology* 1998; **34**: 215–31.

46 Harris Rimmer S, Sawer M. Neoliberalism and gender equality policy in Australia. *Australian Journal of Political Science* 2016; **51**: 742–58.

47 Weller S, O'Neill P. An argument with neoliberalism: Australia's place in a global imaginary. *Dialogues in Human Geography* 2014; **4**: 105–30.

48 Weatherley R. From entitlement to contract: reshaping the welfare state in Australia. *Journal of Sociology and Social Welfare* 1994; **21**: 153–73.

49 Mendes P. Neo-liberalism and welfare conditionality in Australia: a critical analysis of the aims and outcomes of compulsory income management programs. *Journal of Australian Political Economy* 2020; **86**: 157–77.

50 Mendes P, Roche S. How do Australian policymakers frame the causes of and policy solutions to poverty? A critical examination of Anti-Poverty Week parliamentary debates from 2012 to 2021. *Australian Journal of Social Issues* 2023; **58**: 592–606.

51 Xu KQ, Payne CF. A growing divide: trends in social inequalities in healthy longevity in Australia, 2001–20. *Population Studies*; Sep 5: 1–20.

52 Productivity Commission. Closing the gap. Annual data compilation report. Canberra, 2023 https://pc.gov.au/closing-the-gap-data.

53 Evans A. *Changing trends in mortality: an international comparison: 2000 to 2016.* London: Office for National Statistics, 2018 https://www.ons. gov.uk/peoplepopulationandcommunity/birthsdeathsandmarriages/lifee xpectancies/articles/changingtrendsinmortalityaninternationalcompari son/2000to2016.

54 Nusselder WJ, De Waegenaere AMB, Melenberg B, Lyu P, Rubio Valverde JR. Future trends of life expectancy by education in the Netherlands. *BMC Public Health* 2022; **22**: 1664.

55 Butera C. Dutch pension age increase stalled due to life expectancy dip. Chief Investment Officer. 2018; published online 5 Nov. https://www. ai-cio.com/news/dutch-pension-age-increase-stalled-due-life-expecta ncy-dip/.

56 Ortiz I, Cummins M, Capaldo J, Karunanethy K. *The decade of adjustment: a review of austerity trends 2010–2020 in 187 countries.* New York: The South Centre, Columbia University, 2015.

57 Hoekman R, van der Roest J-W, van der Poel H. From welfare state to participation society? Austerity measures and local sport policy in the Netherlands. *International Journal of Sport Policy and Politics* 2018; **10**: 131–46.

58 Hoogenboom M. The Netherlands and the crisis: from activation to 'deficiency compensation'. In: Theodoropoulou S, ed. *Labour market policies in the era of pervasive austerity: a European perspective.* Bristol: Bristol University Press, 2018: 141–68.

59 Janssen D, Jongen W, Schröder-Bäck P. Exploring the impact of austerity-driven policy reforms on the quality of the long-term care provision for older people in Belgium and the Netherlands. *Journal of Aging Studies* 2016; **38**: 92–104.

60 Mody A, Mazzolini G. *Austerity tales: the Netherlands and Italy.* Bruegel. 2014; published online 26 Oct. https://www.bruegel.org/blog-post/austerity-tales-netherlands-and-italy.

61 Steinglass M. Netherlands delays austerity plans. *Financial Times.* 2013; published online 12 April. https://www.ft.com/content/471ead60-a382-11e2-8f9c-00144feabdc0.

62 Bos V, Kunst AE, Keij-Deerenberg IM, Garssen J, Mackenbach JP. Ethnic inequalities in age- and cause-specific mortality in the Netherlands. *International Journal of Epidemiology* 2004; **33**: 1112–19.

63 Bos V, Kunst AE, Garssen J, Mackenbach JP. Socioeconomic inequalities in mortality within ethnic groups in the Netherlands, 1995–2000. *Journal of Epidemiology and Community Health* 2005; **59**: 329.

64 Oudenampsen M, Mellink B. The roots of Dutch frugality: the role of public choice theory in Dutch budgetary policy. *Journal of European Public Policy* 2022; **29**: 1206–24.

65 Agyemang C, Seeleman C, Suurmond J, Stronks K. Racism in health and health care in Europe: where does the Netherlands stand? *European Journal of Public Health* 2007; **17**: 240–1.

66 Gras M, Bovenkerk F. Migrants and ethnic minorities in the Netherlands: discrimination in access to employment. In: Wrench J, Rea A, Ouali N, eds. *Migrants, ethnic minorities and the labour market: integration and exclusion in Europe.* London: Palgrave Macmillan UK, 1999: 93–107.

67 van Heerden S, de Lange SL, van der Brug W, Fennema M. The immigration and integration debate in the Netherlands: discursive and programmatic reactions to the rise of anti-immigration parties. *Journal of Ethnic and Migration Studies 2014;* **40**: 119–36.

68 Rose A. 'Dutch racism is not like anywhere else': refusing color-blind myths in Black feminist otherwise spaces. *Gender & Society* 2022; **36**: 239–63.

69 Bor J, Stokes AC, Raifman J, et al. Missing Americans: early death in the United States – 1933–2021. *PNAS Nexus* 2023; **2**: pgad173.

70 Verguet S, Jamison DT. Improving life expectancy: how many years behind has the USA fallen? A cross-national comparison among high-income countries from 1958 to 2007. *BMJ Open* 2013; **3**: e002814.

71 Woolf SH. Falling behind: the growing gap in life expectancy between the United States and other countries, 1933–2021. *American Journal of Public Health* 2023; **113**: 970 80.

72 Collins C, McCartney G. The impact of neoliberal 'political attack' on health: the case of the 'Scottish effect'. *International Journal of Health Services* 2011; **41**: 501–23.

73 Collins C, McCartney G, Garnham L. Neoliberalism and health inequalities. In: *Health inequalities: critical perspectives*. Oxford: Oxford University Press, 2016: 124–37.

74 Scott-Samuel A, Bambra C, Collins C, Hunter DJ, McCartney G, Smith K. The impact of Thatcherism on health and well-being in Britain. *International Journal of Health Services* 2014; **44**: 53–71.

75 Harriss CL. Successes and failures of President Reagan's economic policies. *Presidential Studies Quarterly* 1984; **14**: 519–25.

76 Modigliani F. Reagan's economic policies: a critique. *Oxford Economic Papers* 1988; **40**: 397–426.

77 Heclo H. The mixed legacies of Ronald Reagan. *Presidential Studies Quarterly* 2008; **38**: 555–74.

78 Meltzer AH. Economic policies and actions in the Reagan administration. *Journal of Post Keynesian Economics* 1988; **10**: 528–40.

79 Muris TJ. Ronald Reagan and the rise of large deficits: what really happened in 1981. *The Independent Review* 2000; **4**: 365–76.

80 Piketty T. *Capital and ideology*. Cambridge, MA: Harvard University Press, 2020.

81 Piketty T, Goldhammer A. *Capital in the twenty-first century*. Cambridge, MA: Harvard University Press, 2014.

82 Krieger N, Rehkopf DH, Chen JT, Waterman PD, Marcelli E, Kennedy M. The fall and rise of US inequities in premature mortality: 1960–2002. *PLOS Medicine* 2008; **5**: e46.

83 Schrecker T, Bambra C. *How politics makes us sick: neoliberal epidemics*. London: Palgrave Macmillan, 2015.

84 Hendi AS. Trends in education-specific life expectancy, data quality, and shifting education distributions: a note on recent research. *Demography* 2017; **54**: 1203–13.

85 Wami W, Walsh D, Hennig BD, et al. Spatial and temporal inequalities in mortality in the USA, 1968–2016. *Health & Place* 2021; **70**: 102586.

86 Dowd JB, Doniec K, Zhang L, Tilstra A. US exceptionalism? International trends in midlife mortality. *medRxiv* 2023; 2023.07.25.23293099.

87 Case A, Deaton A. *Deaths of despair and the future of capitalism.* Princeton: Princeton University Press, 2021.

88 Case A, Deaton A. Rising morbidity and mortality in midlife among white non-Hispanic Americans in the 21st century. *Proceedings of the National Academy of Sciences 2015*; **112**: 15078–83.

89 Woolf SH, Schoomaker H. Life expectancy and mortality rates in the United States, 1959–2017. *JAMA* 2019; **322**: 1996–2016.

90 Harris KM, Majmundar MK, Becker T. *High and rising mortality rates among working-age adults.* Washington, DC: National Academy of Sciences, 2021.

91 Shanahan L, Copeland WE. A deadly drop in rankings: how the United States was left behind in global life expectancy trends. *American Journal of Public Health* 2023; **113**: 961–3.

92 Remington PL. Trends in US life expectancy: falling behind and failing to act. *American Journal of Public Health* 2023; **113**: 956–8.

93 Konings M. Neoliberalism and the American State. *Critical Sociology* 2010; **36**: 741–65.

94 Galea S, Ahern J, Karpati A. A model of underlying socioeconomic vulnerability in human populations: evidence from variability in population health and implications for public health. *Social Science & Medicine* 2005; **60**: 2417–30.

95 Woolf SH. The growing influence of state governments on population health in the United States. *JAMA* 2022; **327**: 1331–2.

96 Montez JK, Beckfield J, Cooney JK, et al. US state policies, politics, and life expectancy. *The Milbank Quarterly* 2020; **98**: 668–99.

97 Tanne JH. US spends more than twice as much on health as similar countries for worse outcomes, finds report. *BMJ* 2023; **383**: p2340.

98 Rovner J. The complicated, political, expensive, seemingly eternal US healthcare debate explained. *BMJ* 2019; **367**: l5885.

99 Kenney GM, McMorrow S, Zuckerman S, Goin DE. A decade of health care access declines for adults holds implications for changes in the Affordable Care Act. *Health Affairs* 2012; **31**: 899–908.

100 Papanicolas I, Woskie LR, Jha AK. Health care spending in the United States and other high-income countries. *JAMA* 2018; **319**: 1024–39.

101 Shrank WH, Rogstad TL, Parekh N. Waste in the US health care system: estimated costs and potential for savings. *JAMA* 2019; **322**: 1501–9.

102 Murray MJ. The pharmaceutical industry: a study in corporate power. *International Journal of Health Services* 1974; **4**: 625–40.

103   Elliot C. *White coat, black hat: adventures on the dark side of medicine.* Boston, MA: Beacon Press, 2014.

104   Relman AS. The new medical-industrial complex. *New England Journal of Medicine* 1980; **303**: 963–70.

105   Fazekas M, Tóth IJ. From corruption to state capture: a new analytical framework with empirical applications from Hungary. *Political Research Quarterly* 2016; **69**: 320–34.

106   Wouters OJ. Lobbying expenditures and campaign contributions by the pharmaceutical and health product industry in the United States, 1999–2018. *JAMA Internal Medicine* 2020; **180**: 688–97.

107   McGreal C. How big pharma's money – and its politicians – feed the US opioid crisis. *The Guardian.* 2017; published online 19 Oct. https://www.theguardian.com/us-news/2017/oct/19/big-pharma-money-lobbying-us-opioid-crisis.

108   Gorodensky A, Kohler JC. State capture through indemnification demands? Effects on equity in the global distribution of COVID-19 vaccines. *Journal of Pharmaceutical Policy and Practice* 2022; **15**: 50.

109   Wray CM, Khare M, Keyhani S. Access to care, cost of care, and satisfaction with care among adults with private and public health insurance in the US. *JAMA Network Open* 2021; **4**: e2110275–e2110275.

110   Wilper AP, Woolhandler S, Lasser KE, McCormick D, Bor DH, Himmelstein DU. Health insurance and mortality in US adults. *American Journal of Public Health* 2009; **99**: 2289–95.

111   Semega J, Kollar M. *Income in the United States: 2021.* Washington, DC: United States Census Bureau, 2022.

112   *Fair taxes on America's billionaires and giant corporations would provide $252 billion in revenue per year to help slash poverty and reduce hunger in the US.* Boston, MA: Oxfam America, 2022 https://www.oxfamamerica.org/press/fair-taxes-on-americas-billionaires-and-giant-corporations-would-provide-252-billion-in-revenue-per-year-to-help-slash-poverty-and-reduce-hunger-in-the-us/.

113   Beckfield J, Bambra C. Shorter lives in stingier states: social policy shortcomings help explain the US mortality disadvantage. *Social Science & Medicine* 2016; **171**: 30–8.

114   Woolf SH, Masters RK, Aron LY. Effect of the COVID-19 pandemic in 2020 on life expectancy across populations in the USA and other high income countries: simulations of provisional mortality data. *BMJ* 2021; **373**: n1343.

115   Krieger N. Discrimination and health inequities. *International Journal of Health Services* 2014; **44**: 643–710.

116 Krieger N. ENOUGH: COVID-19, structural racism, police brutality, plutocracy, climate change – and time for health justice, democratic governance, and an equitable, sustainable future. *American Journal of Public Health* 2020; **110**: 1620–3.

117 Krieger N, Chen JT, Coull BA, Beckfield J, Kiang MV, Waterman PD. Jim Crow and premature mortality among the US Black and white population, 1960–2009: An Age–Period–Cohort Analysis. *Epidemiology* 2014; **25**. https://journals.lww.com/epidem/fulltext/2014/07000/jim_crow_and_premature_mortality_among_the_us.5.aspx.

118 Krieger N, Chen JT, Coull B, Waterman PD, Beckfield J. The unique impact of abolition of Jim Crow laws on reducing inequities in infant death rates and implications for choice of comparison groups in analyzing societal determinants of health. *American Journal of Public Health* 2013; **103**: 2234–44.

119 Bobo LD. Racism in Trump's America: reflections on culture, sociology, and the 2016 US presidential election. *The British Journal of Sociology* 2017; **68**: S85–104.

120 Ruisch BC, Ferguson MJ. Changes in Americans' prejudices during the presidency of Donald Trump. *Nature Human Behaviour* 2022; **6**: 656–65.

121 Ho JY. The contemporary American drug overdose epidemic in international perspective. *Population and Development Review* 2019; **45**: 7–40.

122 Mehta NK, Abrams LR, Myrskylä M. US life expectancy stalls due to cardiovascular disease, not drug deaths. *Proceedings of the National Academy of Sciences 2020;* **117**: 6998–7000.

123 Preston SH, Stokes A. Contribution of obesity to international differences in life expectancy. *American Journal of Public Health* 2011; **101**: 2137–43.

124 Rochel de Camargo K. An alarming trend in US population health. *American Journal of Public Health* 2023; **113**: 952–3.

125 Bishop K. What cuts? US austerity 'tougher than in Europe'. *CNBC Europe*. 2013; published online 15 Nov. https://www.cnbc.com/2013/11/15/what-cuts-us-austerity-tougher-than-in-europe.html.

126 BER Staff. The American austerity playbook. *Berkeley Economic Review*. 2021; published online 4 March. https://econreview.berkeley.edu/the-american-austerity-playbook/.

127 Mattei C. The US debt–ceiling 'deal' was a giant exercise in bipartisan class warfare. *The Guardian*. 2023; published online 14 June.

128 Bambra C. Health inequalities and welfare state regimes: theoretical insights on a public health 'puzzle'. *Journal of Epidemiology and Community Health* 2011; **65**: 740.

129   Bambra C. Going beyond The three worlds of welfare capitalism: regime theory and public health research. *Journal of Epidemiology and Community Health* 2007; **61**: 1098.

130   Kennedy M. *Without a net. Middle class and homeless (with kids) in America: my story*. New York: Viking, 2005.

131   Varoufakis Y. *Adults in the room: my battle with Europe's deep establishment*. London: Bodley Head, 2017.

132   Rajmil L, Hjern A, Spencer N, Taylor-Robinson D, Gunnlaugsson G, Raat H. Austerity policy and child health in European countries: a systematic literature review. *BMC Public Health* 2020; **20**: 564.

133   Stuckler D, Basu S. *The body economic: why austerity kills*. New York: Basic Books, 2013.

134   Stuckler D, Basu S. *The body economic: eight experiments in economic recovery, from Iceland to Greece*. London: Penguin, 2014.

135   Wade RH, Sigurgeirsdottir S. Iceland's rise, fall, stabilisation and beyond. *Cambridge Journal of Economics* 2012; **36**: 127–44.

136   Johnsen G. *Bringing down the banking system: lessons from Iceland*. London: Palgrave Macmillan, 2014.

137   Helgason MS. The 'corporate Vikings': robber barons and corporate raiders. The Reykjavik Grapevine 2010. https://walkthecrash.files. wordpress.com/2015/07/3-grapevine_10_2010-10-corporate-viki ngs.pdf.

138   Tan G. The 10 year recovery, and lessons from Iceland. *Asia & the Pacific Policy Society*. 2018; published online 15 Jan. https://www.poli cyforum.net/10-year-recovery-lessons-iceland/.

139   The true cost of austerity and inequality. Case study: Iceland. Oxfam. 2013; published online Sept. https://www.theeconomyjournal.eu/ texto-diario/mostrar/1336225/the-true-cost-of-austerity-and-inequal ity-case-study-iceland.

140   Gunnlaugsson G. Child health in Iceland before and after the economic collapse in 2008. *Archives of Disease in Childhood* 2016; **101**: 489.

141   Júlíusson ÁD. Inspired by Iceland … no, really! Reykjavik Grapevine. 2011; published online 7 Oct. https://grapevine.is/mag/articles/2011/ 10/07/inspired-by-iceland-no-really/.

142   Árni DJ. Wave of protest. Reykjavik Grapevine. 2011; published online 22 Nov. https://grapevine.is/mag/articles/2011/11/22/wave- of-protest/.

143   England P. Iceland's 'pots and pans revolution': Lessons from a nation that people power helped to emerge from its 2008 crisis all the stronger. Independent. 2015; published online 29 June. https://www.independ ent.co.uk/news/world/europe/iceland-s-pots-and-pans-revolution- lessons-from-a-nation-that-people-power-helped-to-emerge-from- its-2008-crisis-all-the-stronger-10351095.html.

144 Gustafsdottir SS, Fenger K, Halldorsdottir S, Bjarnason T. Social justice, access and quality of healthcare in an age of austerity: users' perspective from rural Iceland. *International Journal of Circumpolar Health* 2017; **76**: 1347476.

145 Stefánsson KH, Arnardóttir L, Karlsson AÖ. Children's deprivation and economic vulnerability in Iceland 2009 and 2014. *Child Indicators Research* 2018; **11**: 783–803.

146 Chzhen Y. Unemployment, social protection spending and child poverty in the European Union during the great recession. *Journal of European Social Policy* 2017; **27**: 123–37.

147 Gunnlaugsson G, Einarsdóttir J. 'All's well in Iceland?' Austerity measures, labour market initiatives, and health and well-being of children. *Nordisk välfärdsforskning | Nordic Welfare Research* 2016; **1**: 30–42.

148 Kentikelenis A, Karanikolos M, Reeves A, McKee M, Stuckler D. Greece's health crisis: from austerity to denialism. *The Lancet* 2014; **383**: 748–53.

149 Nikiforos M. *Crisis, austerity, and fiscal expenditure in Greece: recent experience and future prospects in the post-COVID era.* Annandale-on-Hudson, NY: Levy Economics Institute of Bard College, 2020.

150 Kinsella S. Is Ireland really the role model for austerity? *Cambridge Journal of Economics* 2012; **36**: 223–35.

151 Hespanha P. Health system reforms in southern Europe: crises and alternatives. In: *Policies and social risks in Brazil and Europe: convergences and divergences.* Rio de Janeiro: Hucitec Editora, 2017: 81–110.

152 Teague P. Ireland and the 'GIPS' countries. In: Roche WK, O'Connell PJ, Prothero A, eds. *Austerity and recovery in Ireland: Europe's poster child and the great recession.* Oxford: Oxford University Press, 2016: 141–59. https://doi.org/10.1093/acprof:oso/9780198792376.003.0008.

153 Matsaganis M. *The Greek crisis: social impact and policy responses.* Berlin: Friedrich–Ebert–Stiftung, 2013.

154 Karanikolos M, Kentikelenis A. Health inequalities after austerity in Greece. *International Journal for Equity in Health* 2016; **15**: 83.

155 Paraskevis D, Nikolopoulos G, Tsiara C, et al. HIV-1 outbreak among injecting drug users in Greece, 2011: a preliminary report. *Eurosurveillance* 2011; **16**. DOI: https://doi.org/10.2807/ese.16.36.19962-en.

156 Alexopoulos EC. HIV infections and injecting drug users in Greece. *The Lancet* 2013; **382**: 1095.

157 Rachiotis G, Stuckler D, McKee M, Hadjichristodoulou C. What has happened to suicides during the Greek economic crisis? Findings from an ecological study of suicides and their determinants (2003–2012). *BMJ Open* 2015; **5**: e007295.

158 Branas CC, Kastanaki AE, Michalodimitrakis M, et al. The impact of economic austerity and prosperity events on suicide in Greece: a 30-year interrupted time-series analysis. *BMJ Open* 2015; **5**: e005619.

159 Turley G, McNena S, Robbins G. Austerity and Irish local government expenditure since the great recession. *Administration* 2018; **66**: 1–24.

160 Honohan P, Walsh B. Catching up with the leaders: the Irish hare. *Brookings Papers on Economic Activity* 2002; **2002**: 1–57.

161 Riain SÓ. The road to austerity In: Roche WK, O'Connell PJ, Prothero A, eds. *Austerity and recovery in Ireland: Europe's poster child and the great recession.* Oxford: Oxford University Press 2016: 23–39. https://doi.org/10.1093/acprof:oso/9780198792376.003.0002.

162 Roche WK, O'Connell PJ, Prothero A, eds. *Austerity and recovery in Ireland: Europe's poster child and the great recession.* Oxford: Oxford University Press 2016. https://doi.org/10.1093/acprof:oso/978019 8792376.001.0001.

163 Hanley D. Austerity Ireland: the failure of Irish capitalism. *Journal of Contemporary European Studies* 2015; **23**: 297–8.

164 Boyle R. Public service reform. In: Roche WK, O'Connell PJ, Prothero A, eds. *Austerity and recovery in Ireland: Europe's poster child and the great recession.* Oxford: Oxford University Press, 2016: 214–31. https://doi.org/10.1093/acprof:oso/9780198792376.003.0012.

165 Kinsella S. Economic and fiscal policy. In: Roche WK, O'Connell PJ, Prothero A, eds. *Austerity and recovery in Ireland: Europe's poster child and the great recession.* Oxford: Oxford University Press, 2016: 40–61. https://doi.org/10.1093/acprof:oso/9780198792376.003.0003.

166 Forde C. Community development, policy change, and austerity in Ireland. In: Todd S, Drolet JL, eds. *Community practice and social development in social work.* Singapore: Springer Singapore, 2020: 345–61.

167 O'Rourke P. Austerity and the Irish non-profit voluntary and community sector. In: Baines D, Cunningham I, eds. *Working in the context of austerity: challenges and struggles.* Bristol: Policy Press, 2020: 0.

168 van Lanen S. Living austerity urbanism: space–time expansion and deepening socio-spatial inequalities for disadvantaged urban youth in Ireland. *Urban Geography* 2017; **38**: 1603–13.

169 Kiernan F. What price austerity – a nation's health? The effect of austerity on access to health care in Ireland. *European Journal of Public Health* 2014; **24**: cku165–110.

170 Mercille J, Murphy E. The neoliberalization of Irish higher education under austerity. *Critical Sociology* 2017; **43**: 371–87.

171 Gaynor N. Governing austerity in Dublin: rationalization, resilience, and resistance. *Journal of Urban Affairs* 2020; **42**: 75–90.

172 O'Connell PJ. Unemployment and labour market policy. In: Roche WK, O'Connell PJ, Prothero A, eds. *Austerity and recovery in Ireland: Europe's poster child and the great recession.* Oxford: Oxford University Press, 2016: 232–51. https://doi.org/10.1093/acprof:oso/9780198792376.003.0013.

173 Glynn I, O'Connell PJ. Migration. In: Roche WK, O'Connell PJ, Prothero A, eds. *Austerity and recovery in Ireland: Europe's poster child and the great recession.* Oxford: Oxford University Press, 2016: 290–310. https://doi.org/10.1093/acprof:oso/9780198792376.003.0016.

174 Honohan P. Debt and austerity: post-crisis lessons from Ireland. *Journal of Financial Stability* 2016; **24**: 149–57.

175 Lynch K, Cantillon S, Crean M. Inequality. In: Roche WK, O'Connell PJ, Prothero A, eds. *Austerity and recovery in Ireland: Europe's poster child and the great recession.* Oxford: Oxford University Press, 2016: 252–71. https://doi.org/10.1093/acprof:oso/9780198792376.003.0014.

176 Allen K, O'Boyle B. *Austerity Ireland: the failure of Irish capitalism.* London: Pluto press, 2013.

177 Coffey S. Resources available for public services: how does Ireland compare now and how might we prepare for the future? In: *Debating Austerity in Ireland: Crisis, Experience and Recovery.* Dublin: Royal Irish Academy, 2017.

178 *Health in Ireland: key trends in 2019.* Dublin: Department of Health, 2019.

179 Corcoran P, Griffin E, Arensman E, Fitzgerald AP, Perry IJ. Impact of the economic recession and subsequent austerity on suicide and self-harm in Ireland: an interrupted time series analysis. *International Journal of Epidemiology* 2015; **44**: 969–77.

180 Akram T. The Japanese economy: stagnation, recovery, and challenges. *Journal of Economic Issues* 2019; **53**: 403–10.

181 Wilkinson R, Pickett K. *The spirit level: why equality is better for everyone.* London: Penguin, 2010.

182 Abdul Karim S, Eikemo TA, Bambra C. Welfare state regimes and population health: integrating the East Asian welfare states. *Health Policy* 2010; **94**: 45–53.

183 Shin K-Y. A new approach to social inequality: inequality of income and wealth in South Korea. *The Journal of Chinese Sociology* 2020; **7**: 17.

184 Hall SM, Pimlott-Wilson H, Horton J. *Austerity across Europe: lived experiences of economic crises.* Abingdon: Routledge, 2022.

185 Taylor-Gooby P, Leruth B, Chung H. *After austerity: welfare state transformation in Europe after the great recession.* Oxford: Oxford University Press, 2017.

Moira

1 The success of the strategy can be measured in different ways. Various analyses of the British Social Attitudes Survey showed a changing – and much more negative – view of people in receipt of social security benefits over time.[1] In addition, and arguably in recognition of these changes to public opinion, opposition politicians were observed using similar language: Ed Miliband (then leader of the Labour Party) talked about 'strivers' (thereby differentiating them from the 'skivers' of the UK government's narrative (reference 2), while Rachel Reeves made various statements to reflect a harsher attitude to those in need of help from the state, stating, for example (in 2013), that Labour would be 'tougher' than the Conservatives on welfare reform (reference 3), and in 2015 that Labour were 'not the party of people on benefits' (reference 4).

2 Park A, Clery E, Curtice J, Phillips M, Utting D. British Social Attitudes: the 29th report. London: NatCen Social Research, 2012 https://bsa.natcen.ac.uk/media/1138/bsa29_key_findings.pdf.

3 BBC News. Miliband: Labour united against 'tax on strivers'. BBC. 2013; published online 8 Jan. https://www.bbc.co.uk/news/av/uk-politics-20947675.

4 Helm T. Labour will be tougher than Tories on benefits, promises new welfare chief. *The Guardian*. 2013; published online 12 Oct. https://www.theguardian.com/politics/2013/oct/12/labour-benefits-tories-labour-rachel-reeves-welfare.

5 Gentleman A. Labour vows to reduce reliance on food banks if it comes to power. *The Guardian*. 2015; published online 17 March. https://www.theguardian.com/society/2015/mar/17/labour-vows-to-reduce-reliance-on-food-banks-if-it-comes-to-power.

6 Briant E, Watson N, Philo G. Reporting disability in the age of austerity: the changing face of media representation of disability and disabled people in the United Kingdom and the creation of new 'folk devils'. *Disability & Society* 2013; **28**: 874–89.

7 Mullen A. Media performance in the 'age of austerity': British newspaper coverage of the 2008 financial crisis and its aftermath, 2008–2010. *Journalism* 2021; **22**: 993–1011.

8 Baumberg B, Bell K, Gaffney D, Deacon R, Hood C, Sage D. Benefits stigma in Britain. London: Turn2Us and University of Kent, 2023 https://www.turn2us.org.uk/T2UWebsite/media/Documents/Benefits-Stigma-in-Britain.pdf.

9 Gavin NT. Below the radar: A UK benefit fraud media coverage tsunami: impact, ideology, and society. *British Journal of Sociology* 2021; **72**: 707–24.

10 Monbiot G. Skivers and strivers: this 200-year-old myth won't die. *The Guardian*. 2015; published online 23 June. https://www.theguardian.com/commentisfree/2015/jun/23/skivers-strivers-200-year-old-myth-wont-die.

11   Scottish Government. Welfare Reform (Further Provision) (Scotland) Act 2012: annual report 2017. Edinburgh: Scottish Government, 2017.

12   Coote A, Lyall S. Mythbusters: *'Strivers v. skivers: the workless are worthless'*. London: New Economics Foundation, 2013.

13   Butler P. 'My mother's death was hastened by long delay in processing her benefits'. *The Guardian*. 2015; published online 27 Aug. https://www.theguardian.com/society/2015/aug/27/my-mothers-death-was-hastened-by-long-delay-in-processing-her-benefits.

14   Drury N. Personal communication. 2023.

15   Beatty C, Fothergill S. Welfare reform in the United Kingdom 2010–16: expectations, outcomes, and local impacts. *Social Policy & Administration* 2018; **52**: 950–68.

16   Beatty C, Fothergill S. *The uneven impact of welfare reform: the financial losses to places and people*. Sheffield: Sheffield Hallam, 2016.

17   *The Guardian* newspaper quotes the content of the letter to Moira as stating: 'You requested a mandatory reconsideration of this decision on the grounds that … you were not well and had diarrhoea and that you have diabetes and epilepsy. Having considered all the available evidence, I am unable to accept that a good cause has been shown for not attending the medical assessment.'

Chapter 5

1   Doyle AC. The adventure of Silver Blaze. In: *The Memoirs of Sherlock Holmes*. London: George Newnes, 1893.

2   We note here that we have competing interests, having both worked for public health agencies during this time, with personal responsibilities to describe and explain life expectancy trends. Our approach here is not to seek to defend our own actions or inactions during this period (although we have been the subject of relevant criticism – see Dorling D. The Scottish mortality crisis. *The Geographer* 2016; Summer: 8–9), or to blame individuals, but to identify and expose the systemic reasons for these failures such that they can be avoided in the future. That said, a key reason for writing this book is that this failure is ongoing despite our best efforts, and the evidence requires a broader audience.

3   In the UK, vital event statistics (births and deaths) are generally published in August for the previous year. The time lag is to allow registration of deaths where legal processes are required to establish the cause of death. Even then, the data for each calendar year is usually amended in subsequent years as more accurate estimates of the total population size become available (for example, using census data to adjust the population for the impacts of migration), and to correct for late registrations.

4   The higher mortality in the winter is often attributed to greater infectious disease or greater exposure to cold weather. However, it is also likely to have deeper causes relating to the suitability and affordability of housing, as well as the distribution of and exposure to all of the social determinants of health.

5   Bell DNF, Blanchflower DG. Underemployment in the UK in the great recession. *National Institute Economic Review* 2011; **215**: R23–33.

6   Konzelmann S, Gray M, Donald B. Introduction to the Cambridge Journal of Economics, Cambridge Journal of Regions, Economy and Society and Contributions to Political Economy virtual special issue on assessing austerity. *Cambridge Journal of Economics; Cambridge Journal of Regions, Economy and Society; Contributions to Political Economy.* https://static.primary.prod.gcms.the-infra.com/static/site/cje/document/Introduction-to-Austerity-virtual-issue.pdf?node=1ac8f46a7d82786951e2&version=439045:71d6a5a02b3c73513e2b.

7   Beatty C, Fothergill S. Welfare reform in the United Kingdom 2010–16: expectations, outcomes, and local impacts. *Social Policy & Administration* 2018; **52**: 950–68.

8   Margerison-Zilko C, Goldman-Mellor S, Falconi A, Downing J. Health impacts of the great recession: a critical review. *Current Epidemiology Reports* 2016; **3**: 81–91.

9   Stuckler D, Basu S. *The body economic: why austerity kills.* New York: Basic Books, 2013.

10 Stuckler D, Basu S. *The body economic: eight experiments in economic recovery, from Iceland to Greece.* London: Penguin, 2014.

11 Stuckler D, Reeves A, Karanikolos M, McKee M. The health effects of the global financial crisis: can we reconcile the differing views? A network analysis of literature across disciplines. *Health Economics, Policy and Law* 2015; **10**: 83–99.

12 Catalano R, Goldman-Mellor S, Saxton K, et al. The health effects of economic decline. *Annual Review of Public Health* 2011; **32**: 431–50.

13 Rachiotis G, Stuckler D, McKee M, Hadjichristodoulou C. What has happened to suicides during the Greek economic crisis? Findings from an ecological study of suicides and their determinants (2003–2012). *BMJ Open* 2015; **5**: e007295.

14 Antonakakis N, Collins A. The impact of fiscal austerity on suicide mortality: evidence across the 'eurozone periphery'. *Social Science & Medicine* 2015; **145**: 63–78.

15 Corcoran P, Griffin E, Arensman E, Fitzgerald AP, Perry IJ. Impact of the economic recession and subsequent austerity on suicide and self-harm in Ireland: an interrupted time series analysis. *International Journal of Epidemiology* 2015; **44**: 969–77.

16   Varoufakis Y. *Adults in the room: my battle with Europe's deep establishment.*
London: Bodley Head, 2017.

17   McKee M, Karanikolos M, Belcher P, Stuckler D. Austerity: a failed
experiment on the people of Europe. *Clinical Medicine* 2012; **12**: 346.

18   Marmot M, Allen J, Goldblatt P, et al. *Fair society, healthy lives: Marmot
review report.* London: Institute of Health Equity.

19   Commission on the Social Determinants of Health. *Closing the gap in
a generation: health equity through action on the social determinants of health.*
Geneva: WHO, 2008.

20   Beeston C, McCartney G, Ford J, et al. *Health inequalities policy review
for the Scottish Ministerial Task Force on Health Inequalities.* Glasgow: NHS
Health Scotland, 2013 http://www.healthscotland.scot/media/1053/
1-healthinequalitiespolicyreview.pdf.

21   McCartney G, Hearty W, Arnot J, Popham F, Cumbers A, McMaster R.
Impact of political economy on population health: a systematic review
of reviews. *American Journal of Public Health* 2019; **109**: e1–12.

22   *Inequalities in health: report of a working group chaired by Sir Douglas Black.*
London: Department of Health and Social Security, 1980.

23   Whitehead M. *The health divide.* London: Pelican Books, 1988.

24   Walsh D, McCartney G, Collins C, Taulbut M, Batty GD. History,
politics and vulnerability: explaining excess mortality in Scotland and
Glasgow. *Public Health* 2017; **151**: 1–12.

25   Paraskevis D, Nikolopoulos G, Tsiara C, et al. HIV-1 outbreak among
injecting drug users in Greece, 2011: a preliminary report. *Eurosurveillance*
2011; **16**. DOI: https://doi.org/10.2807/ese.16.36.19962-en.

26   Reeves A, Basu S, McKee M, Marmot M, Stuckler D. Austere or not?
UK coalition government budgets and health inequalities. *Journal of the
Royal Society of Medicine* 2013; **106**: 432–6.

27   Garthwaite K. Fear of the brown envelope: exploring welfare reform
with long-term sickness benefits recipients. *Social Policy & Administration*
2014; **48**: 782–98.

28   Kentikelenis A, Karanikolos M, Reeves A, McKee M, Stuckler D.
Greece's health crisis: from austerity to denialism. *The Lancet* 2014;
383: 748–53.

29   Kiernan F. What price austerity – a nation's health? The effect of austerity
on access to health care in Ireland. *European Journal of Public Health* 2014;
24: cku165-110.

30   Taylor-Robinson D, Whitehead M, Barr B. Great leap backwards. *BMJ*
2014; **349**: g7350.

31   Mølbak K, Espenhain L, Nielsen J, et al. Excess mortality among the
elderly in European countries, December 2014 to February 2015.
Eurosurveillance 2015; **20**. DOI: https://doi.org/10.2807/1560-7917.
ES2015.20.11.21065.

32 Schrecker T, Bambra C. *How politics makes us sick: neoliberal epidemics.* London: Palgrave Macmillan, 2015.

33 Branas CC, Kastanaki AE, Michalodimitrakis M, et al. The impact of economic austerity and prosperity events on suicide in Greece: a 30-year interrupted time-series analysis. *BMJ Open* 2015; **5**: e005619.

34 Barr B, Kinderman P, Whitehead M. Trends in mental health inequalities in England during a period of recession, austerity and welfare reform 2004 to 2013. *Social Science & Medicine* 2015; **147**: 324–31.

35 Loopstra R, Reeves A, Taylor-Robinson D, Barr B, McKee M, Stuckler D. Austerity, sanctions, and the rise of food banks in the UK. *BMJ* 2015; **350**: h1775.

36 Loopstra R, Reeves A, Barr B, Taylor-Robinson D, McKee M, Stuckler D. The impact of economic downturns and budget cuts on homelessness claim rates across 323 local authorities in England, 2004–12. *Journal of Public Health* 2016; **38**: 417–25.

37 Loopstra R, McKee M, Katikireddi SV, Taylor-Robinson D, Barr B, Stuckler D. Austerity and old-age mortality in England: a longitudinal cross-local area analysis, 2007–2013. *Journal of the Royal Society of Medicine* 2016; **109**: 109–16.

38 Janssen D, Jongen W, Schröder-Bäck P. Exploring the impact of austerity-driven policy reforms on the quality of the long-term care provision for older people in Belgium and the Netherlands. *Journal of Aging Studies* 2016; **38**: 92–104.

39 Beckfield J, Bambra C. Shorter lives in stingier states: social policy shortcomings help explain the US mortality disadvantage. *Social Science & Medicine* 2016; **171**: 30–8.

40 Karanikolos M, Kentikelenis A. Health inequalities after austerity in Greece. *International Journal for Equity in Health* 2016; **15**: 83.

41 Reeves A, Clair A, McKee M, Stuckler D. Reductions in the United Kingdom's government housing benefit and symptoms of depression in low-income households. *American Journal of Epidemiology* 2016; **184**: 421–9.

42 Barr B, Taylor-Robinson D, Stuckler D, Loopstra R, Reeves A, Whitehead M. 'First, do no harm': are disability assessments associated with adverse trends in mental health? A longitudinal ecological study. *Journal of Epidemiology and Community Health* 2016; **70**: 339.

43 Barnes MC, Gunnell D, Davies R, et al. Understanding vulnerability to self-harm in times of economic hardship and austerity: a qualitative study. *BMJ Open* 2016; **6**: e010131.

44 Newton J. Re: Sharp spike in deaths in England and Wales needs investigating, says public health expert. *BMJ* 2016; **352**: i981.

45 Watkins J, Wulaningsih W, Da Zhou C, et al. Effects of health and social care spending constraints on mortality in England: a time trend analysis. *BMJ Open* 2017; **7**: e017722.

46 Hiam L, Dorling D, Harrison D, McKee M. What caused the spike in mortality in England and Wales in January 2015? *Journal of the Royal Society of Medicine* 2017; **110**: 131–7.

47 Green MA, Dorling D, Minton J, Pickett KE. Could the rise in mortality rates since 2015 be explained by changes in the number of delayed discharges of NHS patients? *Journal of Epidemiology and Community Health* 2017; **71**: 1068.

48 Garthwaite K, Bambra C. 'How the other half live': lay perspectives on health inequalities in an age of austerity. *Social Science & Medicine* 2017; **187**: 268–75.

49 Cooper V, Whyte D. *The violence of austerity*. London: Pluto Press, 2017.

50 Basu S, Carney MA, Kenworthy NJ. Ten years after the financial crisis: the long reach of austerity and its global impacts on health. *Social Science & Medicine* 2017; **187**: 203–7.

51 Ruckert A, Labonté R. Health inequities in the age of austerity: the need for social protection policies. *Social Science & Medicine* 2017; **187**: 306–11.

52 Saltkjel T, Ingelsrud MH, Dahl E, Halvorsen K. A fuzzy set approach to economic crisis, austerity and public health. Part I. European countries' conformity to ideal types during the economic downturn. *Scandinavian Journal of Public Health* 2017; **45**: 41–7.

53 Saltkjel T, Ingelsrud MH, Dahl E, Halvorsen K. A fuzzy set approach to economic crisis, austerity and public health. Part II: How are configurations of crisis and austerity related to changes in population health across Europe? *Scandinavian Journal of Public Health* 2017; **45**: 48–55.

54 Chzhen Y. Unemployment, social protection spending and child poverty in the European Union during the great recession. *Journal of European Social Policy* 2017; **27**: 123–37.

55 Newton J, Baker A, Fitzpatrick J, Ege F. What's happening with mortality rates in England? 2017; published online 20 July. https://ukhsa.blog.gov.uk/2017/07/20/whats-happening-with-mortality-rates-in-england/.

56 Katikireddi SV, Molaodi OR, Gibson M, Dundas R, Craig P. Effects of restrictions to income support on health of lone mothers in the UK: a natural experiment study. *The Lancet Public Health* 2018; **3**: e333–40.

57 van der Wel KA, Saltkjel T, Chen W-H, Dahl E, Halvorsen K. European health inequality through the 'great recession': social policy matters. *Sociology of Health & Illness* 2018; **40**: 750–68.

58 Green MA. Austerity and the new age of population health? *Scandinavian Journal of Public Health* 2018; **46**: 38–41.

59 Rajmil L, Taylor-Robinson D, Gunnlaugsson G, Hjern A, Spencer N. Trends in social determinants of child health and perinatal outcomes in European countries 2005–2015 by level of austerity imposed by governments: a repeat cross-sectional analysis of routinely available data. *BMJ Open* 2018; **8**: e022932.

60 Mattheys K, Warren J, Bambra C. 'Treading in sand': A qualitative study of the impact of austerity on inequalities in mental health. *Social Policy & Administration* 2018; **52**: 1275–89.

61 Prayogo E, Chater A, Chapman S, et al. Who uses foodbanks and why? Exploring the impact of financial strain and adverse life events on food insecurity. *Journal of Public Health* 2018; **40**: 676–83.

62 Thomson RM, Niedzwiedz CL, Katikireddi SV. Trends in gender and socioeconomic inequalities in mental health following the great recession and subsequent austerity policies: a repeat cross-sectional analysis of the health surveys for England. *BMJ Open* 2018; **8**: e022924.

63 Hiam L, Dorling D. Rise in mortality in England and Wales in first seven weeks of 2018. *BMJ* 2018; **360**. DOI:10.1136/bmj.k1090.

64 Hiam L, Harrison D, McKee M, Dorling D. Why is life expectancy in England and Wales 'stalling'? *Journal of Epidemiology and Community Health* 2018; **72**: 404.

65 Hiam L, Dorling D, McKee M. Rise in mortality – when will the government take note? *BMJ* 2018; **361**: k2747.

66 Baker A, Ege F, Fitzpatrick J, Newton J. Response to articles on mortality in England and Wales. *Journal of the Royal Society of Medicine* 2018; **111**: 40–1.

67 Raleigh VS. Stalling life expectancy in the UK. *BMJ* 2018; **362**: k4050.

68 Raleigh V. *Stalling life expectancy in the UK*. London: The King's Fund, 2018 https://www.kingsfund.org.uk/publications/stalling-life-expectancy-uk.

69 *A review of recent trends in mortality in England*. London: Public Health England, 2018.

70 Dorling D. Austerity bites: falling life expectancy in the UK. 2019; published online 19 March. https://blogs.bmj.com/bmj/2019/03/19/danny-dorling.

71 Ryan F. *Crippled: austerity and the demonization of disabled people*. London: Verso, 2019.

72 Cheetham M, Moffatt S, Addison M, Wiseman A. Impact of Universal Credit in north east England: a qualitative study of claimants and support staff. *BMJ Open* 2019; **9**: e029611.

73 Loopstra R, Reeves A, Tarasuk V. The rise of hunger among low-income households: an analysis of the risks of food insecurity between 2004 and 2016 in a population-based study of UK adults. *Journal of Epidemiology & Community Health* 2019; **73**: 668–73.

74 Rajmil L, Fernández de Sanmamed M-J. Austerity policies and mortality rates in European countries, 2011–2015. *American Journal of Public Health* 2019; **109**: 768–70.

75 Toffolutti V, Suhrcke M. Does austerity really kill? *Economics & Human Biology* 2019; **33**: 211–23.

76 Murphy M, Luy M, Torrisi O. *Stalling of mortality in the United Kingdom and Europe: an analytical review of the evidence*. London: London School of Economics, 2019.

77 Marshall L, Finch D, Cairncross L, Bibby J. *Mortality and life expectancy trends in the UK: stalling progress*. London: Health Foundation, 2019.

78 Montez JK, Beckfield J, Cooney JK, et al. US state policies, politics, and life expectancy. *The Milbank Quarterly* 2020; **98**: 668–99.

79 Krieger N. ENOUGH: COVID-19, structural racism, police brutality, plutocracy, climate change – and time for health justice, democratic governance, and an equitable, sustainable future. *American Journal of Public Health* 2020; **110**: 1620–3.

80 Wickham S, Bentley L, Rose T, Whitehead M, Taylor-Robinson D, Barr B. Effects on mental health of a UK welfare reform, Universal Credit: a longitudinal controlled study. *The Lancet Public Health* 2020; **5**: e157–64.

81 Rajmil L, Hjern A, Spencer N, Taylor-Robinson D, Gunnlaugsson G, Raat H. Austerity policy and child health in European countries: a systematic literature review. *BMC Public Health* 2020; **20**: 564.

82 Prędkiewicz P, Bem A, Siedlecki R, Kowalska M, Robakowska M. An impact of economic slowdown on health. New evidence from 21 European countries. *BMC Public Health* 2022; **22**: 1405.

83 Ploetner C, Telford M, Brækkan K, et al. Understanding and improving the experience of claiming social security for mental health problems in the west of Scotland: a participatory social welfare study. *Journal of Community Psychology* 2020; **48**: 675–92.

84 Marmot M, Allen J, Boyce T, Goldblatt P, Morrison J. *Health Equity in England: The Marmot Review 10 years on*. London: Institute of Health Equity, 2020.

85 Public Health Wales. *Life Expectancy and Mortality in Wales (2020)*. Cardiff: Public Health Wales, 2020 https://phw.nhs.wales/services-and-teams/observatory/data-and-analysis/life-expectancy-and-mortality-in-wales-2020/.

86 *Is cardiovascular disease slowing improvements in life expectancy? OECD and the King's Fund workshop proceedings*. Paris: OECD, 2020.

87 Richardson E, Taulbut M, Robinson M, Pulford A, McCartney G. The contribution of changes to tax and social security to stalled life expectancy trends in Scotland: a modelling study. *Journal of Epidemiology and Community Health* 2021; **75**: 365.

88   Alexiou A, Fahy K, Mason K, et al. Local government funding and life expectancy in England: a longitudinal ecological study. *The Lancet Public Health* 2021; **6**: e641–7.

89   Martin S, Longo F, Lomas J, Claxton K. Causal impact of social care, public health and healthcare expenditure on mortality in England: cross-sectional evidence for 2013/2014. *BMJ Open* 2021; **11**: e046417.

90   Cherrie M, Curtis S, Baranyi G, et al. A data linkage study of the effects of the great recession and austerity on antidepressant prescription usage. *European Journal of Public Health* 2021; **31**: 297–303.

91   Simpson J, Albani V, Bell Z, Bambra C, Brown H. Effects of social security policy reforms on mental health and inequalities: a systematic review of observational studies in high-income countries. *Social Science & Medicine* 2021; **272**: 113717.

92   Koltai J, McKee M, Stuckler D. Association between disability-related budget reductions and increasing drug-related mortality across local authorities in Great Britain. *Social Science & Medicine* 2021; **284**: 114225.

93   Jenkins RH, Aliabadi S, Vamos EP, et al. The relationship between austerity and food insecurity in the UK: a systematic review. *eClinicalMedicine* 2021; **33**. DOI:10.1016/j.eclinm.2021.100781.

94   Mason KE, Alexiou A, Bennett DL, Summerbell C, Barr B, Taylor-Robinson D. Impact of cuts to local government spending on Sure Start children's centres on childhood obesity in England: a longitudinal ecological study. *Journal of Epidemiology and Community Health* 2021; **75**: 860.

95   Hiam L, Dorling D, McKee M. Austerity, not influenza, caused the UK's health to deteriorate. Let's not make the same mistake again. *Journal of Epidemiology and Community Health* 2021; **75**: 312.

96   *Chief Medical Officer for Scotland: annual report 2020–2021.* Edinburgh: Scottish Government, 2021 https://www.gov.scot/publications/cmo-annual-report-2020-21/documents/.

97   Reeves A, Fransham M, Stewart K, Patrick R. Does capping social security harm health? A natural experiment in the UK. *Social Policy & Administration* 2022; **56**: 345–59.

98   Stokes J, Bower P, Guthrie B, et al. Cuts to local government spending, multimorbidity and health-related quality of life: a longitudinal ecological study in England. *The Lancet Regional Health – Europe* 2022; **19**. DOI:10.1016/j.lanepe.2022.100436.

99   Roscoe S, Pryce R, Buykx P, Gavens L, Meier PS. Is disinvestment from alcohol and drug treatment services associated with treatment access, completions and related harm? An analysis of English expenditure and outcomes data. *Drug and Alcohol Review* 2022; **41**: 54–61.

100 Friebel R, Yoo KJ, Maynou L. Opioid abuse and austerity: evidence on health service use and mortality in England. *Social Science & Medicine* 2022; **298**: 114511.

101 Walsh D, Dundas R, McCartney G, Gibson M, Seaman R. Bearing the burden of austerity: how do changing mortality rates in the UK compare between men and women? *Journal of Epidemiology and Community Health* 2022; **76**: 1027.

102 Hall SM, Pimlott-Wilson H, Horton J. *Austerity across Europe: lived experiences of economic crises.* Abingdon: Routledge, 2022.

103 McCartney G, McMaster R, Popham F, Dundas R, Walsh D. Is austerity a cause of slower improvements in mortality in high-income countries? A panel analysis. *Social Science & Medicine* 2022; **313**: 115397.

104 Gschwind L, Ratzmann N, Beste J. Protected against all odds? A mixed-methods study on the risk of welfare sanctions for immigrants in Germany. *Social Policy & Administration* 2022; **56**: 502–17.

105 Woolf SH. The growing influence of state governments on population health in the United States. *JAMA* 2022; **327**: 1331–2.

106 Darlington-Pollock F, Green MA, Simpson L. Why were there 231,707 more deaths than expected in England between 2010 and 2018? An ecological analysis of mortality records. *Journal of Public Health* 2022; **44**: 310–18.

107 Sosenko F, Bramley G, Bhattacharjee A. Understanding the post-2010 increase in food bank use in England: new quasi-experimental analysis of the role of welfare policy. *BMC Public Health* 2022; **22**: 1363.

108 Kim C, Teo C, Nielsen A, Chum A. What are the mental health consequences of austerity measures in public housing? A quasi-experimental study. *Journal of Epidemiology and Community Health* 2022; **76**: 730.

109 McCartney G, Walsh D, Fenton L, Devine R. *Resetting the course for population health.* Glasgow: Glasgow Centre for Population Health and the University of Glasgow, 2022.

110 Raleigh V. *What is happening to life expectancy in England?* London: The King's Fund, 2022 https://www.kingsfund.org.uk/publications/whats-happening-life-expectancy-england.

111 Fahy K, Alexiou A, Daras K, et al. Mental health impact of cuts to local government spending on cultural, environmental and planning services in England: a longitudinal ecological study. *BMC Public Health* 2023; **23**: 1441.

112 Alexiou A, Mason K, Fahy K, Taylor-Robinson D, Barr B. Assessing the impact of funding cuts to local housing services on drug and alcohol related mortality: a longitudinal study using area-level data in England. *International Journal of Housing Policy* 2023; **23**: 362–80.

113 Mason KE, Alexiou A, Barr B, Taylor-Robinson D. Impact of cuts to local authority spending on cultural, environmental and planning services on inequalities in childhood obesity in England: a longitudinal ecological study. *Health & Place* 2023; **80**: 102999.

114 Lee SC, DelPozo-Banos M, Lloyd K, Jones I, Walters JTR, John A. Trends in socioeconomic inequalities in incidence of severe mental illness: A population-based linkage study using primary and secondary care routinely collected data between 2000 and 2017. *Schizophrenia Research* 2023; **260**: 113–22.

115 Finch D, Wilson H, Bibby J. *Leave no one behind: the state of health and health inequalities in Scotland*. London: The Health Foundation, 2023.

116 Whitty CJM, Smith G, McBride M, Atherton F, Powis SH, Stokes-Lampard H. Restoring and extending secondary prevention. *BMJ* 2023; **380**: p201.

117 Fenton L, Minton J, Ramsay J, et al. Recent adverse mortality trends in Scotland: comparison with other high-income countries. *BMJ Open* 2019; **9**: e029936.

118 Fenton L, Wyper GM, McCartney G, Minton J. Socioeconomic inequality in recent adverse all-cause mortality trends in Scotland. *Journal of Epidemiology and Community Health* 2019; **73**: 971.

119 Pebody RG, Green HK, Warburton F, et al. Significant spike in excess mortality in England in winter 2014/15: influenza the likely culprit. *Epidemiology & Infection* 2018; **146**: 1106–13.

120 Statens Serum Institut. *EuroMOMO*. EuroMOMO. https://www. euromomo.eu/ (accessed 6 Aug 2023).

121 Statens Serum Institut. *FluMOMO*. FluMOMO. https://www.eurom omo.eu/how-it-works/flumomo/ (accessed 6 Aug 2023).

122 Vestergaard LS, Nielsen J, Krause TG, et al. Excess all-cause and influenza-attributable mortality in Europe, December 2016 to February 2017. *Eurosurveillance* 2017; **22**. DOI: https://doi.org/10.2807/1560-7917.ES.2017.22.14.30506.

123 Nielsen J, Vestergaard LS, Richter L, et al. European all-cause excess and influenza-attributable mortality in the 2017/18 season: should the burden of influenza B be reconsidered? *Clinical Microbiology and Infection* 2019; **25**: 1266–76.

124 Office for National Statistics. Spike in number of deaths in 2015 driven by increased mortality in over 75s. 2016; published online 7 April. https://www.ons.gov.uk/news/news/spikeinnumberofdeathsin2015d rivenbyincreasedmortalityinover75s.

125 Fransham M, Dorling D. Have mortality improvements stalled in England? *BMJ* 2017; **357**: j1946.

126 Walsh D, McCartney G. *Changing mortality rates in Scotland and the UK: an updated summary*. Glasgow: Glasgow Centre for Population Health, 2023 https://www.gcph.co.uk/assets/0000/9348/Changing_mortality_ra tes_in_Scotland_and_the_UK_-_an_updated_summary_FINAL.pdf.

127 Walsh D, McCartney G, Minton J, Parkinson J, Shipton D, Whyte B. Changing mortality trends in countries and cities of the UK: a population-based trend analysis. *BMJ Open* 2020; **10**: e038135.

128 *Mortality trends UK-wide workshops*. Edinburgh: ScotPHO https://www. scotpho.org.uk/population-dynamics/stalling-mortality-trends/resour ces-and-key-references/ (accessed 20 Aug 2023).

129 Minton J, Fletcher E, Ramsay J, Little K, McCartney G. How bad are life expectancy trends across the UK, and what would it take to get back to previous trends? *Journal of Epidemiology and Community Health* 2020; **74**: 741.

130 McCartney G, Leyland A, Walsh D, Ruth D. Scaling COVID-19 against inequalities: should the policy response consistently match the mortality challenge? *Journal of Epidemiology and Community Health* 2021; **75**: 315.

131 The authors of this book were leaders of ScotPHO throughout the relevant time period, and we are aware that this gives us a particular perspective on the contributions of the organisations we discuss here. Up until 2020, ScotPHO staff were mainly situated with NHS Health Scotland (HS) and the Information Services Division (ISD) of NHS National Services Scotland, with a smaller contribution from the Glasgow Centre for Population Health (GCPH). In April 2020, HS and ISD were brought together into Public Health Scotland, along with Health Protection Scotland (HPS).

132 Dorling D. The Scottish mortality crisis. *The Geographer* 2016; Summer: 8–9.

133 This group was the Scottish Mortality Special Interest Group, administered by the Scottish Public Health Network (ScotPHN), and involving public health expertise from across national and local health boards, the Scottish Government, the Glasgow Centre for Population Health (GCPH), and National Records of Scotland (NRS).

134 McCartney G, Douglas M, Taulbut M, Katikireddi SV, McKee M. Tackling population health challenges as we build back from the pandemic. *BMJ* 2021; **375**: e066232.

135 Walsh D, Wyper GMA, McCartney G. Trends in healthy life expectancy in the age of austerity. *Journal of Epidemiology and Community Health* 2022; **76**: 743.

136 The ScotPHO website (https://www.scotpho.org.uk/population-dynam ics/stalling-mortality-trends/) provided an up-to-date forum from 2017 onwards for analysis and briefings of the changed trends in Scotland.

137 The three national public health functions prior to April 2020 in Scotland were: NHS Health Scotland, the Information and Statistics Division (ISD) of NHS National Services Scotland, and Health Protection Scotland (a unit of NHS National Services Scotland).

138 Currie J, Schilling HT, Evans L, et al. Contribution of avoidable mortality to life expectancy inequalities in Wales: a decomposition by age and by cause between 2002 and 2020. *Journal of Public Health* 2022; published online Nov. DOI: 10.1093/pubmed/fdac133.

139 Atcheson R, Carson M, Laverty C. *Life expectancy in Northern Ireland 2019–21*. Belfast: Department of Health, 2023 https://www.health-ni.gov.uk/sites/default/files/publications/health/hscims-life-expectancy-ni-2019-21.pdf.

140 World Health Statistics 2023. Geneva: World Health Organisation, 2023.

141 Dwyer-Lindgren L, Kendrick P, Kelly YO, et al. Life expectancy by county, race, and ethnicity in the USA, 2000–19: a systematic analysis of health disparities. *The Lancet* 2022; **400**: 25–38.

142 Good Law Project. *Tufton Street: shine a light on dark money in politics.* https://goodlawproject.org/case/tufton-street-shine-a-light-on-dark-money-in-politics/ (accessed 20 Aug 2023).

143 Boseley S. Austerity blamed for life expectancy stalling for first time in century. *The Guardian.* 2020; published online 25 Feb. https://www.theguardian.com/society/2020/feb/24/austerity-blamed-for-life-expectancy-stalling-for-first-time-in-century.

144 Minton J, Hiam L, McKee M, Dorling D. Slowing down or returning to normal? Life expectancy improvements in Britain compared to five large European countries before the COVID-19 pandemic. *British Medical Bulletin* 2022; **145**: 6–16.

145 Hiam L, Dorling D, McKee M. When experts disagree: interviews with public health experts on health outcomes in the UK 2010–2020. *Public Health* 2023; **214**: 96–105.

146 Wang H, Abbas KM, Abbasifard M, et al. Global age-sex-specific fertility, mortality, healthy life expectancy (HALE), and population estimates in 204 countries and territories, 1950–2019: a comprehensive demographic analysis for the Global Burden of Disease Study 2019. *The Lancet* 2020; **396**: 1160–203.

147 Kelly-Irving M, Ball WP, Bambra C, et al. Falling down the rabbit hole? Methodological, conceptual and policy issues in current health inequalities research. *Critical Public Health* 2023; **33**: 37–47.

148 Smith KE, Kandlik Eltanani M. What kinds of policies to reduce health inequalities in the UK do researchers support? *Journal of Public Health* 2015; **37**: 6–17.

149 Smith KE, Bambra C, Hill SE. *Health inequalities: critical perspectives.* Oxford: Oxford University Press, 2015.

150 Strassheim H, Kettunen P. When does evidence-based policy turn into policy-based evidence? Configurations, contexts and mechanisms. *Evidence & Policy* 2014; **10**: 259–77.

151 Marmot MG. Evidence based policy or policy based evidence? *BMJ* 2004; **328**: 906.

152 McCartney G, Collins C, Dorling D. Would action on health inequalities have saved New Labour? *BMJ* 2010; **340**: c3294.

153 McCartney G, Garnham L, Gunson D, Collins C. When do your politics become a competing interest? *BMJ* 2011; **342**: d269.

154 Krieger N. *Ecosocial theory, embodied truths, and the people's health*, 1st edition. New York: Oxford University Press, 2021.

155 Krieger N. *Epidemiology and the people's health. Theory and context*. Oxford: Oxford University Press, 2011.

156 Beckfield J, Krieger N. Epi + demos + cracy: linking political systems and priorities to the magnitude of health inequities – evidence, gaps, and a research agenda. *Epidemiologic Reviews* 2009; **31**: 152–77.

157 McCartney G, Collins C, Mackenzie M. What (or who) causes health inequalities: theories, evidence and implications? *Health Policy* 2013; **113**: 221–7.

158 Tannahill A. Beyond evidence – to ethics: a decision-making framework for health promotion, public health and health improvement. *Health Promotion International* 2008; **23**: 380–90.

159 Olin Wright E. *Understanding class*. London: Verso, 2015.

160 Friel S, Townsend B, Fisher M, Harris P, Freeman T, Baum F. Power and the people's health. *Social Science & Medicine* 2021; **282**: 114173.

161 McCartney G, Dickie E, Escobar O, Collins C. Health inequalities, fundamental causes and power: towards the practice of good theory. *Sociology of Health & Illness* 2021; **43**: 20–39.

162 This is generally true in parliamentary democracies such as the UK, but there are exceptions. For example, unelected members of the House of Lords in the UK can be appointed to ministerial positions, as happened in November 2023 with the appointment of David Cameron to the House of Lords, and to the role of Foreign Secretary.

163 Diethelm P, McKee M. Denialism: what is it and how should scientists respond? *European Journal of Public Health* 2009; **19**: 2–4.

164 McKee M, Diethelm P. How the growth of denialism undermines public health. *BMJ* 2010; **341**: c6950.

165 Dorries N. 2020; published online 28 Jan. https://hansard.parliament.uk/Commons/2020-01-28/debates/BFC8A790-4102-4512-B1FC-084CCCB3F7B9/LifeExpectancy.

166 Philp C. *Economic situation*. London: Hansard, 2022 https://hansard. parliament.uk/Commons/2022-10-12/debates/5CCA11C4-441D-4CDC-8C1C-8B53E882966A/EconomicSituation?highlight=thewl iss#contribution-231A05B6-A9DF-4DBB-934C-13118BE27098.

167 Osborne G. George Osborne's speech to the Conservative party conference in full. *The Guardian*. 2010; published online 4 Oct. https:// www.theguardian.com/politics/2010/oct/04/george-osborne-spe ech-conservative-conference.

168 Doyle-Price J. 2018; published online 18 April. https://hansard.parliam ent.uk/Commons/2018-04-18/debates/6AEE73CE-7C3C-4DC0-A8EB-DA7FE45A34EE/AusterityLifeExpectancy.

169 Hammond S. 2019; published online 25 April. https://hansard.par liament.uk/Commons/2019-04-25/debates/3C3AF91B-23A9-4419-A104-34A8261A4F88/Women%E2%80%99SLifeExpectancy.

170 Courts R. 2018; published online 18 April. https://hansard.parliam ent.uk/Commons/2018-04-18/debates/6AEE73CE-7C3C-4DC0-A8EB-DA7FE45A34EE/AusterityLifeExpectancy.

171 Selous A. 2018; published online 18 April. https://hansard.parliam ent.uk/Commons/2018-04-18/debates/6AEE73CE-7C3C-4DC0-A8EB-DA7FE45A34EE/AusterityLifeExpectancy.

172 Marmot M. Twitter. 2023; published online 20 June. https://twitter. com/MichaelMarmot/status/1671250131872800769.

173 McKee M. Twitter. 2023; published online 20 June. https://twitter. com/TheBMA/status/1671169694173364225.

174 General Medical Council. *The duties of a doctor registered with the General Medical Council*. London: General Medical Council, 2023 https:// www.gmc-uk.org/ethical-guidance/ethical-guidance-for-doctors/ good-medical-practice/duties-of-a-doctor.

Ellen

1 Leshner AI. Addiction is a brain disease, and it matters. *Science* 1997; **278**: 45–7.

2 Walsh D, McCartney G, Minton J, Parkinson J, Shipton D, Whyte B. Deaths from 'diseases of despair' in Britain: comparing suicide, alcohol-related and drug-related mortality for birth cohorts in Scotland, England and Wales, and selected cities. *Journal of Epidemiology and Community Health* 2021; **75**: 1195.

3 Parkinson J, Minton J, Lewsey J, Bouttell J, McCartney G. Drug-related deaths in Scotland 1979–2013: evidence of a vulnerable cohort of young men living in deprived areas. *BMC Public Health* 2018; **18**: 357.

4 *Problem drug use in Scotland: Government response to the Committee's First Report of Session 2019*. London: UK Parliament Scottish Affairs Committee https://publications.parliament.uk/pa/cm5801/cmselect/cmscotaf/698/69802.htm.

5 *Problem drug use in Scotland. London: UK Parliament Scottish Affairs Committee*, 2019 https://publications.parliament.uk/pa/cm201919/cmselect/cmscotaf/44/4402.htm.

6 The 142 per cent figure is based on the comparison between the age-standardised mortality rates in the periods 2010/12 and 2019/21. Three-year averages are used to 'smooth' the data, and overcome the issue of particular 'spikes' of deaths in certain years. The 10,435 is the total number of drug-related deaths recorded by the National Records of Scotland between 2010 and 2021.

7 *Drug-related deaths in Scotland in 2022*. Edinburgh: National Records of Scotland, 2022 https://www.nrscotland.gov.uk/statistics-and-data/statistics/statistics-by-theme/vital-events/deaths/drug-related-deaths-in-scotland/2022.

Chapter 6

1 Tucker M. *The thick of it. Season 3, Episode 1*. London: BBC, 2009.

2 McCartney G, Walsh D, Fenton L, Devine R. *Resetting the course for population health*. Glasgow: Glasgow Centre for Population Health and the University of Glasgow, 2022.

3 Douglas M, Katikireddi SV, Taulbut M, McKee M, McCartney G. Mitigating the wider health effects of covid-19 pandemic response. *BMJ* 2020; **369**: m1557.

4 Douglas M, McCartney G, Richardson E, Taulbut M, Craig N. *Population health impacts of the rising cost of living in Scotland: a rapid health impact assessment*. Edinburgh: Public Health Scotland, 2022 https://publichealthscotland.scot/publications/population-health-impacts-of-the-rising-cost-of-living-in-scotland-a-rapid-health-impact-assessment/population-health-impacts-of-the-rising-cost-of-living-in-scotland-a-rapid-health-impact-assessment/.

5 Richardson E, McCartney G, Taulbut M, Douglas M, Craig N. Population mortality impacts of the rising cost of living in Scotland: scenario modelling study. *BMJ Public Health* 2023; **1**: e000097.

6 Broadbent P, Thomson R, Kopasker D, et al. The public health implications of the cost-of-living crisis: outlining mechanisms and modelling consequences. *The Lancet Regional Health – Europe* 2023; **27**. DOI: 10.1016/j.lanepe.2023.100585.

7 McCartney G, Douglas M, Taulbut M, Katikireddi SV, McKee M. Tackling population health challenges as we build back from the pandemic. *BMJ* 2021; **375**: e066232.

8   Di Angelantonio E, Bhupathiraju SN, Wormser D, et al. Body-mass index and all-cause mortality: individual-participant-data meta-analysis of 239 prospective studies in four continents. *The Lancet* 2016; **388**: 776–86.

9   BMI for each person is calculated as weight (in kilograms) divided by the square of height (in metres).

10 BMI is useful for tracking population trends in excess weight, but it has flaws. First, it is not easily applicable to children and young people. Second, not all causes of excess weight are necessarily unhealthy – such as from pregnancy or musculature. Third, a decrease in BMI is not necessarily healthy, as it can be caused by illnesses such as cancer or under-nutrition.

11 Malik VS, Willet WC, Hu FB. Nearly a decade on: trends, risk factors and policy implications in global obesity. *Nature Reviews Endocrinology* 2020; **16**: 615–16.

12 Butland B, Jebb S, Kopelman P, et al. *Tackling obesities: future choices – project report*. London: Foresight, UK Government, 2007.

13 Sumińska M, Podgórski R, Bogusz-Górna K, Skowrońska B, Mazur A, Fichna M. Historical and cultural aspects of obesity: from a symbol of wealth and prosperity to the epidemic of the 21st century. *Obesity Reviews* 2022; **23**: e13440.

14 Hoebel J, Kuntz B, Kroll LE, et al. Socioeconomic inequalities in the rise of adult obesity: a time-trend analysis of national examination data from Germany, 1990–2011. *Obesity Facts* 2019; **12**: 344–56.

15 *Health survey for England 2018*. London: Office for National Statistics, 2019.

16 *Scottish health survey 2019 – volume 1: main report*. Edinburgh: Scottish Government, 2020 https://www.gov.scot/publications/scottish-hea lth-survey-2019-volume-1-main-report/pages/5/.

17 Reyes Matos U, Mesenburg MA, Victora CG. Socioeconomic inequalities in the prevalence of underweight, overweight, and obesity among women aged 20–49 in low- and middle-income countries. *International Journal of Obesity* 2020; **44**: 609–16.

18 Fryar CD, Carroll MD, Afful J. *Prevalence of overweight, obesity, and severe obesity among adults aged 20 and over: United States, 1960–1962 through 2017–2018*. National Center for Health Statistics, 2020.

19 Walsh D, Tod E, McCartney G, Levin KA. How much of the stalled mortality trends in Scotland and England can be attributed to obesity? *BMJ Open* 2022; **12**: e067310.

20 Swinburn B, Egger G, Raza F. Dissecting obesogenic environments: the development and application of a framework for identifying and prioritizing environmental interventions for obesity. *Preventive Medicine* 1999; **29**: 563–70.

21 Dolega L, Reynolds J, Singleton A, Pavlis M. Beyond retail: new ways of classifying UK shopping and consumption spaces. *Environment and Planning B: Urban Analytics and City Science* 2021; **48**: 132–50.

22 Understanding Glasgow – *The Glasgow Indicators Project: transport trends.* Glasgow: Glasgow Centre for Population Health, 2023 https://www.understandingglasgow.com/indicators/transport/travel_to_work/trends/scottish_trends.

23 Aldred R, Verlinghieri E, Sharkey M, Itova I, Goodman A. Equity in new active travel infrastructure: a spatial analysis of London's new low traffic neighbourhoods. *Journal of Transport Geography* 2021; 96 : 103194.

24 Ryde GC, Brown HE, Gilson ND, Brown WJ. Are we chained to our desks? Describing desk-based sitting using a novel measure of occupational sitting. *Journal of Physical Activity and Health* 2014; **11**: 1318–23.

25 Gutierrez A, Guzman NG, Ramos R, Uylengco JKA. The empirical change of playing habits among children. *International Journal of Multidisciplinary: Applied Business and Education Research* 2022; **3**: 303–17.

26 Holt NL, Neely KC, Spence JC, et al. An intergenerational study of perceptions of changes in active free play among families from rural areas of Western Canada. *BMC Public Health* 2016; **16**: 829.

27 Watchman T, Spencer-Cavaliere N. Times have changed: parent perspectives on children's free play and sport. *Psychology of Sport and Exercise* 2017; **32**: 102–12.

28 McQuade L, McLaughlin M, Giles M, Cassidy T. Play across the generations: perceptions of changed play patterns in childhood. *Journal of Social Sciences and Humanities* 2019; **5**: 90–6.

29 Gilmore AB, Fabbri A, Baum F, et al. Defining and conceptualising the commercial determinants of health. *The Lancet* 2023; **401**: 1194–213.

30 Stuckler D, McKee M, Ebrahim S, Basu S. Manufacturing epidemics: the role of global producers in increased consumption of unhealthy commodities including processed foods, alcohol, and tobacco. *PLOS Medicine* 2012; **9**: e1001235.

31 Schrecker T, Bambra C. Obesity: how politics makes us fat. In: Schrecker T, Bambra C, eds. *How politics makes us sick: neoliberal epidemics.* London: Palgrave Macmillan UK, 2015: 23–41.

32 Douglas M. *Health and transport: a guide.* Edinburgh: Scottish Health and Inequality Impact Assessment Network (SHIIAN), 2018.

33 Douglas MJ, Watkins SJ, Gorman DR, Higgins M. Are cars the new tobacco? *Journal of Public Health* 2011; **33**: 160–9.

34 Costa-Font J, Mas N. 'Globesity'? The effects of globalization on obesity and caloric intake. *Food Policy* 2016; **64**: 121–32.

35 Kickbusch I, Piselli D, Agrawal A, et al. The Lancet and Financial Times commission on governing health futures 2030: growing up in a digital world. *The Lancet* 2021; **398**: 1727–76.

36 Kickbusch I, Demaio S, Grimes A, Williams C, de Leeuw E, Herriot M. The wellbeing economy is within reach – let's grasp it for better health. *Health Promotion International* 2022; **37**: daac055.

37 The Social Dilemma. Netflix, 2020 https://www.thesocialdilemma.com/.

38 This method of estimation uses 'population attributable fractions'. In this way of estimating causes, contributions overlap because multiple causes can sit on the same pathway. This means that a comprehensive assessment of causes usually adds up to much more than 100 per cent.

39 Preston SH, Stokes A. Contribution of obesity to international differences in life expectancy. *American Journal of Public Health* 2011; **101**: 2137–43.

40 Gorman E, Leyland AH, McCartney G, et al. Adjustment for survey non-representativeness using record-linkage: refined estimates of alcohol consumption by deprivation in Scotland. *Addiction* 2017; **112**: 1270–80.

41 WHO. *WHO statement regarding cluster of pneumonia cases in Wuhan, China.* WHO Western Pacific Hong Kong SAR (China), 2020 https://www.who.int/hongkongchina/news/detail/09-01-2020-who-statement-regarding-cluster-of-pneumonia-cases-in-wuhan-china.

42 *The true death toll of COVID-19: estimating global excess mortality.* Geneva: WHO, 2021 https://www.who.int/data/stories/the-true-death-toll-of-covid-19-estimating-global-excess-mortality.

43 *COVID-19: epidemiology, virology and clinical features.* London: UK Health Security Agency, 2022 https://www.gov.uk/government/publications/wuhan-novel-coronavirus-background-information/wuhan-novel-coronavirus-epidemiology-virology-and-clinical-features#:~:text=Disease%20course%20and%20clinical%20features,-The%20incubation%20period&text=COVID%2D19%20presents%20with%20a,ageusia%20(loss%20of%20taste).

44 Bambra C, Marmot M. *Expert report for the UK COVID-19 public inquiry. Module 1: health inequalities.* London: UK Covid-19 Public Inquiry, 2023 https://covid19.public-inquiry.uk/documents/inq000195843-expert-report-by-professor-clare-bambra-and-professor-sir-michael-marmot-dated-30-may-2023/.

45 Bambra C, Lynch J, Smith KE. *The unequal pandemic: COVID-19 and health inequalities.* Bristol: Policy Press, 2021.

46 Bambra C, Riordan R, Ford J, Matthews F. The COVID-19 pandemic and health inequalities. *Journal of Epidemiology and Community Health* 2020; **74**: 964.

47 Krieger N. ENOUGH: COVID-19, structural racism, police brutality, plutocracy, climate change – and time for health justice, democratic governance, and an equitable, sustainable future. *American Journal of Public Health* 2020; **110**: 1620–3.

48 Foundational Economy Collective. *Foundational economy: the infrastructure of everyday life.* Manchester: Manchester University Press, 2018.

49 Abbasi K. COVID-19: Social murder, they wrote – elected, unaccountable, and unrepentant. *BMJ* 2021; **372**: n314.

50 Brauner JM, Mindermann S, Sharma M, et al. Inferring the effectiveness of government interventions against COVID-19. *Science* 2021; **371**: eabd9338.

51 Meyerowitz-Katz G, Bhatt S, Ratmann O, et al. Is the cure really worse than the disease? The health impacts of lockdowns during COVID-19. *BMJ Global Health* 2021; **6**: e006653.

52 Hanlon P, Chadwick F, Shah A, et al. COVID-19? Exploring the implications of long-term condition type and extent of multimorbidity on years of life lost: a modelling study [version 3; peer review: 3 approved]. *Wellcome Open Research* 2021; **5**. DOI: 10.12688/wellcomeopenres.15849.3.

53 Wang H, Abbas KM, Abbasifard M, et al. Global age-sex-specific fertility, mortality, healthy life expectancy (HALE), and population estimates in 204 countries and territories, 1950–2019: a comprehensive demographic analysis for the Global Burden of Disease Study 2019. *The Lancet* 2020; **396**: 1160–203.

54 Gao M, Piernas C, Astbury NM, et al. Associations between body-mass index and COVID-19 severity in 6.9 million people in England: a prospective, community-based, cohort study. *The Lancet Diabetes & Endocrinology* 2021; **9**: 350–9.

55 Moynihan R, Sanders S, Michaleff ZA, et al. Impact of COVID-19 pandemic on utilisation of healthcare services: a systematic review. *BMJ Open* 2021; **11**: e045343.

56 Goyal DK, Mansab F, Naasan AP, et al. Restricted access to the NHS during the COVID-19 pandemic: is it time to move away from the rationed clinical response? *The Lancet Regional Health – Europe* 2021; **8**. DOI: 10.1016/j.lanepe.2021.100201.

57 Harrison D. What is driving all cause excess mortality? *BMJ* 2022; **376**: o100.

58 Yasin YJ, Grivna M, Abu-Zidan FM. Global impact of COVID-19 pandemic on road traffic collisions. *World Journal of Emergency Surgery* 2021; **16**: 51.

59 Raleigh V. What is driving excess deaths in England and Wales? *BMJ* 2022; **379**: o2524.

60 Caul S. *International comparisons of possible factors affecting excess mortality.* London: Office for National Statistics, 2022 https://www.ons.gov.uk/peoplepopulationandcommunity/healthandsocialcare/healthandwellbeing/articles/internationalcomparisonsofpossiblefactorsaffectingexcessmortality/2022-12-20.

61 Whitty CJM, Smith G, McBride M, Atherton F, Powis SH, Stokes-Lampard H. Restoring and extending secondary prevention. *BMJ* 2023; **380**: p201.

62 McCartney G, Walsh D. Rapid response to: restoring and extending secondary prevention. *BMJ* 2023; **380**: p201.

63 Green L, Ashton K, Bellis M, Clements T, Douglas M. Predicted and observed impacts of COVID-19 lockdowns: two health impact assessments in Scotland and Wales. *Health Promotion International* 2022; **37**: daac134.

64 McCartney G, McMaster R, Popham F, Dundas R, Walsh D. Is austerity a cause of slower improvements in mortality in high-income countries? A panel analysis. *Social Science & Medicine* 2022; **313**: 115397.

65 McGowan VJ, Bambra C. COVID-19 mortality and deprivation: pandemic, syndemic, and endemic health inequalities. *The Lancet Public Health* 2022; **7**: e966–75.

66 Richardson E, Fenton L, Parkinson J, et al. The effect of income-based policies on mortality inequalities in Scotland: a modelling study. *The Lancet Public Health* 2020; **5**: e150–6.

67 Richardson E, Taulbut M, Robinson M, Pulford A, McCartney G. The contribution of changes to tax and social security to stalled life expectancy trends in Scotland: a modelling study. *Journal of Epidemiology and Community Health* 2021; **75**: 365.

68 IPCC. *Climate change 2022: impacts, adaptation, and vulnerability. Contribution of Working Group II to the Sixth Assessment Report of the Intergovernmental Panel on Climate Change.* Intergovernmental Panel on Climate Change (IPCC), 2022.

69 Romanello M, Di Napoli C, Drummond P, et al. The 2022 report of the Lancet Countdown on health and climate change: health at the mercy of fossil fuels. *The Lancet* 2022; **400**: 1619–54.

70 McCartney G, Leyland A, Walsh D, Ruth D. Scaling COVID-19 against inequalities: should the policy response consistently match the mortality challenge? *Journal of Epidemiology and Community Health* 2021; **75**: 315.

71 Walsh D, McCartney G. *Changing mortality rates in Scotland and the UK: an updated summary.* Glasgow: Glasgow Centre for Population Health, 2023 https://www.gcph.co.uk/assets/0000/9348/Changing_mortality_rates_in_Scotland_and_the_UK_-_an_updated_summary_FINAL.pdf.

David

1 Gentleman A. 'No one should die penniless and alone': the victims of Britain's harsh welfare sanctions. *The Guardian*. 2014; published online 3 Aug. https://www.theguardian.com/society/2014/aug/03/victims-brita ins-harsh-welfare-sanctions.

2 Webster D. *Briefing: benefit sanctions statistics*. London: Child Poverty Action Group, 2023 https://cpag.org.uk/policy-and-campaigns/brief ing/david-webster-university-glasgow-briefings-benefit-sanctions.

3 Kennedy S, Hobson F, Mackley A, Kirk-Wade E, Lewis A. *Department for Work and Pensions policy on benefit sanctions*. London: House of Commons Library, 2022 https://commonslibrary.parliament.uk/research-briefings/cdp-2022-0230/.

4 UK Government. *Welfare Reform Act 2012*. London: The Stationery Office, 2012 https://www.legislation.gov.uk/ukpga/2012/5/pdfs/ukpga_20120005_en.pdf.

5 Three main changes were introduced in 2012: the scope of sanctions and conditionality were considerably extended; the length of sanctions was increased; and the concept of 'escalating sanctions' was introduced.

6 Thompson G. Personal communication. 2023.

Chapter 7

1 Thunberg G. Speech at UN Climate Change COP24 Conference. 2018; published online Dec. https://www.youtube.com/watch?v=VFkQSGyeCWg.

2 Engels F. *The condition of the working class in England*. Oxford: Oxford University Press, 2009.

3 Chakrabortty A. Over 170 years after Engels, Britain is still a country that murders its poor. *The Guardian*. 2017; published online 20 June. https://www.theguardian.com/commentisfree/2017/jun/20/engels-britain-murders-poor-grenfell-tower.

4 'The shift towards austerity [has] also legitimised the use of economic violence against disabled people, and other groups deemed "unproductive" by the ruling class. In the UK ... [it] would not be an exaggeration to describe some of these cases ... as social murder (see reference 7)'

5 Abbasi K. Covid-19: Social murder, they wrote – elected, unaccountable, and unrepentant. *BMJ* 2021; **372**: n314.

6 Medvedyuk S, Govender P, Raphael D. The reemergence of Engels' concept of social murder in response to growing social and health inequalities. *Social Science & Medicine* 2021; **289**: 114377.

7 Blakely G. Capitalism has always been authoritarian. *Tribune*. 2023; published online March. https://tribunemag.co.uk/2021/03/capitalism-has-always-been-authoritarian.

8   In most (but not necessarily absolutely all) cases, you'd hope the brick causes only a very minor injury.

9   Despite introducing of austerity policies which have so clearly widened health inequalities, both the Conservative-Liberal Democrat Coalition government (from 2010), and then the Conservative government (from 2015), have also explicitly emphasised the need to narrow health inequalities. For example, narrowing inequalities in life expectancy and healthy life expectancy were 'overarching' aims laid out in the Coalition's 2012 'Healthy lives, healthy people' report, while similar reductions in healthy life expectancy inequalities are a core component of the Conservative government's 'levelling up' strategy.

10   *Healthy lives, healthy people: improving outcomes and supporting transparency.* London: Department of Health, 2012.

11   *Levelling Up the United Kingdom.* London: UK Government, 2022 https://www.gov.uk/government/publications/levelling-up-the-uni ted-kingdom.

12   Blackman T, Hunter D, Marks L, et al. Wicked comparisons: reflections on cross-national research about health inequalities in the UK. *Evaluation* 2010; **16**: 43–57.

13   Craig P. *Focus on inequalities: a framework for action.* Glasgow: Glasgow Centre for Population Health, 2011.

14   Wistow J, Blackman T, Byrne D, Wistow G. Health inequalities, wicked problems and complexity. In: *Studying health inequalities: an applied approach.* Bristol: Bristol University Press, 2016.

15   Plamondon KM, Pemberton J. Blending integrated knowledge translation with global health governance: an approach for advancing action on a wicked problem. *Health Research Policy and Systems* 2019; **17**: 24.

16   Finch D, Wilson H, Bibby J. *Leave no one behind: the state of health and health inequalities in Scotland.* London: The Health Foundation, 2023.

17   McCartney G, Collins C, Mackenzie M. What (or who) causes health inequalities: theories, evidence and implications? *Health Policy* 2013; **113**: 221–7.

18   Doyal L, Pennell I. *The political economy of health.* London: Pluto Press, 1979.

19   Navarro V. Social class, political power, and the state and their implications in medicine. *International Journal of Health Services* 1977; **7**: 255–92.

20   McCartney G, Hearty W, Arnot J, Popham F, Cumbers A, McMaster R. Impact of political economy on population health: a systematic review of reviews. *American Journal of Public Health* 2019; **109**: e1–12.

21   Clare Bambra. Work, worklessness and the political economy of health inequalities. *Journal of Epidemiology and Community Health* 2011; **65**: 746.

22 Mooney G. *The health of nations: towards a new political economy.* London: Zed Books, 2012.

23 Krieger N. *Epidemiology and the people's health. Theory and context.* Oxford: Oxford University Press, 2011.

24 Marmot M. Social causes of the slowdown in health improvement. *Journal of Epidemiology and Community Health* 2018; **72**: 359.

25 Macintyre S. *Inequalities in health in Scotland: what are they and what can we do about them?* Glasgow: MRC Social & Public Health Sciences Unit, 2007.

26 Beeston C, McCartney G, Ford J, et al. *Health inequalities policy review for the Scottish Ministerial Task Force on Health Inequalities.* Glasgow: NHS Health Scotland, 2013 http://www.healthscotland.scot/media/1053/1-healthinequalitiespolicyreview.pdf.

27 Marmot M, Allen J, Goldblatt P, et al. *Fair society, healthy lives: Marmot review report.* London: Institute of Health Equity.

28 Commission on the Social Determinants of Health. *Closing the gap in a generation: health equity through action on the social determinants of health.* Geneva: WHO, 2008.

29 Sayer A, McCartney G. Economic relationships and health inequalities: improving public health recommendations. *Public Health* 2021; **199**: 103–6.

30 Sayer A. *Why we can't afford the rich.* Bristol: Policy Press, 2014.

31 Walsh D, Lowther M, McCartney G, Reid K. Can Scotland achieve its aim of narrowing health inequalities in a post-pandemic world? *Public Health in Practice* 2020; **1**: 100042.

32 McCartney G, Walsh D, Fenton L, Devine R. *Resetting the course for population health.* Glasgow: Glasgow Centre for Population Health and the University of Glasgow, 2022.

33 Eikemo T, Hoffmann R, Kulik M, et al. *EURO-GBD-SE: the potential for reduction of health inequalities in Europe.* Rotterdam: Erasmus University, 2012.

34 Taulbut M, Walsh D, McCartney G, et al. Spatial inequalities in life expectancy within postindustrial regions of Europe: a cross-sectional observational study. *BMJ Open* 2014; **4**: e004711.

35 Walsh D, McCartney G. *Changing mortality rates in Scotland and the UK: an updated summary.* Glasgow: Glasgow Centre for Population Health, 2023 https://www.gcph.co.uk/assets/0000/9348/Changing_mortality_rates_in_Scotland_and_the_UK_-_an_updated_summary_FINAL.pdf.

36 Friel S, Townsend B, Fisher M, Harris P, Freeman T, Baum F. Power and the people's health. *Social Science & Medicine* 2021; **282**: 114173.

37 McCartney G, Dickie E, Escobar O, Collins C. Health inequalities, fundamental causes and power: towards the practice of good theory. *Sociology of Health & Illness* 2021; **43**: 20–39.

38 Piketty T. *Capital and ideology*. Cambridge, MA: Harvard University Press, 2020.

39 Piketty T. *Capital in the twenty-first century*. Cambridge, MA: The Bellknap Press of Harvard University Press, 2014.

40 Dorling D. *Injustice: why social inequality still persists*. Bristol: Policy Press, 2015.

41 Cumbers A, McMaster R, Cabaço S, White MJ. Reconfiguring economic democracy: generating new forms of collective agency, individual economic freedom and public participation. *Work, Employment and Society* 2020; **34**: 678–95.

42 Tod E, Shipton D, McCartney G, et al. What is the potential for plural ownership to support a more inclusive economy? A systematic review protocol. *Systematic Reviews* 2022; **11**: 76.

43 *What are the principles of a good social security system?* London: Child Poverty Action Group, Undated https://cpag.org.uk/policy-and-campaigns/secure-futures-children-and-families#Principles.

44 OECD. Benefits in unemployment, share of previous income (indicator). 2023; published online Oct. https://data.oecd.org/benwage/benefits-in-unemployment-share-of-previous-income.htm.

45 Esser I, Ferrarini T, Nelson K, Palme J, Sjöberg O. *Unemployment benefits in EU Member States*. Brussels: European Commission, 2013.

46 Waddell G, Burton AK. *Is work good for your health and well-being?* London: The Stationery Office, 2006.

47 Taulbut M, Agbato D, McCartney G. *Working and hurting? Monitoring the health and health inequalities impacts of the economic downturn and changes to the social security system*. Glasgow: NHS Health Scotland, 2018.

48 Stone J. *Local indicators of child poverty after housing costs, 2021/22*. Loughborough: Loughborough University, 2023 https://endchildpoverty.org.uk/wp-content/uploads/2023/06/Local-indicators-of-child-poverty-after-housing-costs_Final-Report-3.pdf.

49 Confusingly, the UK government's so-called 'living wage' is effectively the minimum wage for people aged 21 years or more; different (smaller) pay rates apply to people aged 16–20 years, and these are referred to as the minimum wage for those age bands. These rates are mandatory for employers. In contrast, the value of the higher, Real Living Wage is set each year by the Living Wage Foundation and is voluntary.

50 Living Wage Foundation. https://www.livingwage.org.uk/.

51 Greer SL. Labour politics as public health: how the politics of industrial relations and workplace regulation affect health. *European Journal of Public Health* 2018; **28**: 34–7.

52 *Fair work framework*. Glasgow: Fair Work Convention, 2016 https://www.fairworkconvention.scot/wp-content/uploads/2018/12/Fair-Work-Convention-Framework-PDF-Full-Version.pdf.

53 Chown M (@marcuschown). Smiling Danny Alexander opens a food bank in Inverness. A picture that requires no comment. Twitter/X, 2014 https://twitter.com/marcuschown/status/436905431785811968.

54 Shorrocks A, Davies J, Lluberas R. *Global wealth report 2022*. Zürich: Credit Suisse, 2022 https://www.credit-suisse.com/about-us/en/reports-research/global-wealth-report.html.

55 Sosenko F, Bramley G, Bhattacharjee A. Understanding the post-2010 increase in food bank use in England: new quasi-experimental analysis of the role of welfare policy. *BMC Public Health* 2022; **22** : 1363.

56 Wilkinson P, Smith KR, Beevers S, Tonne C, Oreszczyn T. Energy, energy efficiency, and the built environment. *The Lancet* 2007; **370**: 1175–87.

57 Wilkinson P, Smith KR, Davies M, et al. Public health benefits of strategies to reduce greenhouse-gas emissions: household energy. *The Lancet* 2009; **374**: 1917–29.

58 A 'living rent' is one where social housing rental costs would be linked to the level of local earnings.

59 Butland B, Jebb S, Kopelman P, et al. *Tackling obesities: future choices – project report*. London: Foresight, UK Government, 2007.

60 *The scale of economic inequality in the UK*. London: The Equality Trust, n.d. https://equalitytrust.org.uk/scale-economic-inequality-uk.

61 Anderson H. *UK heading for the biggest overnight cut to the basic rate of social security since World War II*. York: Joseph Rowntree Foundation, 2021 https://www.jrf.org.uk/press/uk-heading-biggest-overnight-cut-basic-rate-social-security-world-war-ii.

62 *Universal Credit – the impact of cutting the £20-a-week*. York: Joseph Rowntree Foundation, 2021 https://www.jrf.org.uk/universal-credit-cut-impact-constituency.

63 Universal Credit cut: everything you need to know. *Citizens Advice*, 2021 https://www.citizensadvice.org.uk/about-us/about-us1/media/press-releases/universal-credit-cut-everything-you-need-to-know/.

64 Spoor E. *The real impact of removing the Universal Credit uplift*. London: The Trussell Trust, 2021 https://www.trusselltrust.org/2021/02/08/the-real-impact-of-removing-the-universal-credit-uplift/.

65 Iacobucci G. COVID-19: government writes off £10bn on unusable, overpriced, or undelivered PPE. *BMJ* 2022; **376**: o296.

66 Dyer C. COVID-19: government's use of VIP lane for awarding PPE contracts was unlawful, says judge. *BMJ* 2022; **376**: o96.

67 Ferguson NM, Laydon D, Nedjati-Gilani G, et al. *Impact of non-pharmaceutical interventions (NPIs) to reduce COVID-19 mortality and healthcare demand*. London: Imperial College, 2020.

68 McCartney G, Leyland A, Walsh D, Ruth D. Scaling COVID-19 against inequalities: should the policy response consistently match the mortality challenge? *Journal of Epidemiology and Community Health* 2021; **75**: 315.

69 Bradshaw J. *Why the two-child policy is the worst social security policy ever.* London: Social Policy Association, 2017 https://social-policy.org.uk/50-for-50/two-child-policy/.

70 Watson I. Two-child benefit cap: Keir Starmer to face challenge from Labour policy body. *BBC News.* 2023; published online 18 July. https://www.bbc.co.uk/news/uk-politics-66231718.

71 Butler P. Labour MPs attack Starmer's commitment to keep Tories' two-child benefit limit. *The Guardian.* 2023; published online 17 July. https://www.theguardian.com/politics/2023/jul/17/labour-mps-keir-starmer-tories-two-child-benefit-limit.

Appendix

1 Angrist JD, Pischke J-S. *Mostly harmless econometrics: an empiricist's companion.* Princeton: Princeton University Press, 2009.

2 Angrist JD, Pischke J-S. *Mastering metrics: the path from cause to effect.* Princeton: Princeton University Press, 2014.

3 Huntington-KIein N. *The effect: an introduction to research design and causality.* Abingdon: CRC Press, 2022.

4 Cunningham S. *Causal inference: the mixtape.* New Haven, CT: Yale University Press, 2020.

5 Lawlor DA, Tilling K, Davey Smith G. Triangulation in aetiological epidemiology. *International Journal of Epidemiology* 2016; **45**: 1866–86.

6 Munafò MR, Davey Smith G. Repeating experiments is not enough. *Nature* 2018; **553**: 399–401.

7 Skivington K, Matthews L, Simpson SA, et al. A new framework for developing and evaluating complex interventions: update of Medical Research Council guidance. *BMJ* 2021; **374**: n2061.

8 Shimonovich M, Pearce A, Thomson H, Keyes K, Katikireddi SV. Assessing causality' in epidemiology: revisiting Bradford Hill to incorporate developments in causal thinking. *European Journal of Epidemiology* 2021; **36**: 873–87.

9 Alexiou A, Fahy K, Mason K, et al. Local government funding and life expectancy in England: a longitudinal ecological study. *The Lancet Public Health* 2021; **6**: e641–7.

10 Beckfield J, Bambra C. Shorter lives in stingier states: social policy shortcomings help explain the US mortality disadvantage. *Social Science & Medicine* 2016; **171**: 30–8.

11 Loopstra R, McKee M, Katikireddi SV, Taylor-Robinson D, Barr B, Stuckler D. Austerity and old-age mortality in England: a longitudinal cross-local area analysis, 2007–2013. *Journal of the Royal Society of Medicine* 2016; **109**: 109–16.

12 Martin S, Longo F, Lomas J, Claxton K. Causal impact of social care, public health and healthcare expenditure on mortality in England: cross-sectional evidence for 2013/2014. *BMJ Open* 2021; **11**: e046417.

13 McCartney G, McMaster R, Popham F, Dundas R, Walsh D. Is austerity a cause of slower improvements in mortality in high-income countries? A panel analysis. *Social Science & Medicine* 2022; **313**: 115397.

14 Prędkiewicz P, Bem A, Siedlecki R, Kowalska M, Robakowska M. An impact of economic slowdown on health. New evidence from 21 European countries. *BMC Public Health* 2022; **22**: 1405.

15 Rajmil L, Fernández de Sanmamed M-J. Austerity policies and mortality rates in European countries, 2011–2015. *American Journal of Public Health* 2019; **109**: 768–70.

16 Seaman R, Walsh D, Beatty C, McCartney G, Dundas R. Social security cuts and life expectancy: a longitudinal analysis of local authorities in England, Scotland and Wales. *Journal of Epidemiology and Community Health* 2023; **78**: jech-2023-220328.

17 Note that this paper does not claim causality, as the editors of the journal insisted on this being taken out throughout – despite it using causal methods – reflecting a deep reluctance within parts of the public health community to say something is causal even when the methods allow that inference to be made.

18 Toffolutti V, Suhrcke M. Does austerity really kill? *Economics & Human Biology* 2019; **33**: 211–23.

19 Watkins J, Wulaningsih W, Da Zhou C, et al. Effects of health and social care spending constraints on mortality in England: a time trend analysis. *BMJ Open* 2017; **7**: e017722.

Index

References to figures and tables appear in *italic* type. References to endnotes show both the page number and the note number (178n8).